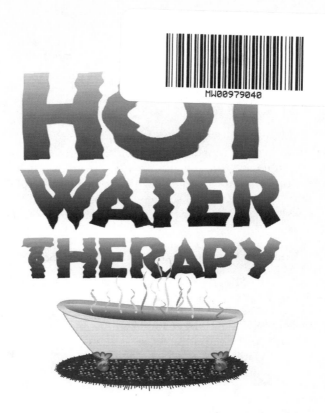

HOT
WATER
THERAPY

By Dr. Patrick Horay and David Harp

NEW HARBINGER PUBLICATIONS, INC.

Publisher's Note

This publication is designed to provide accurate and authoritative information in regard to the subject matter covered. It is sold with the understanding that the publisher is not engaged in rendering chiropractic, legal, or medical services. If expert assistance or counseling is needed, the services of a competent professional should be sought.

Library of Congress Catalog Card Number: 91-052838

ISBN 1-879237-06-7 Paperback
ISBN 1-879237-07-5 Hardcover

Copyright © by New Harbinger Publications, Inc.
                5674 Shattuck Avenue
                Oakland, CA 94609

Printed in the United States of America on recycled paper

Cover and illustrations by SHELBY DESIGNS AND ILLUSTRATES
Edited by Nina Sonenberg

1st Printing December, 1991 4,000 copies

*Each patient carries his own doctor inside him.
They come to us not knowing that truth. We are
at our best when we give the doctor who resides
within each patient a chance to work.*

— Dr. Albert Schweitzer

Contents

Introduction   *vii*

1   **About the Method**   *1*

2   **About Hot Water**   *7*

3   **About Your Body**   *15*

4   **Where Does It Hurt?**   *23*

5   **Deep Massage Techniques**   *37*

    A Touch of Relaxation   *39*

    The Finger Walk: Searching for Pressure Points   *40*

    The Finger Stroke: Flushing the Muscle   *42*

    Massage 1: The Trapezius Walk   *44*

    Massage 2: The Sacrum Stroke   *45*

    Massage 3: Using Your BackuPressure Device   *48*

6   **Exercise Techniques**   *51*

    Exercise 1: Shoulder Lifts   *53*

    Exercise 2: Shoulder Circles   *57*

    Exercise 3: Head Rock   *60*

    Exercise 4: Elbow Across Chest   *64*

    Exercise 5: Seal to Swan   *69*

    Exercise 6: Scared Cat to Swaybacked Horse   *72*

    Exercise 7: Knee Walk   *76*

    Exercise 8: Knee Circles   *78*

    Exercise 9: Pelvic Tilt   *80*

7   **Stretching Techniques**   *85*

    Stretch 1: Head to the Side   *87*

    Stretch 2: Head Down   *90*

    Stretch 3: Elbow Across Chest   *92*

    Stretch 4: Arm Over Head   *96*

    Stretch 5: Seal to Swan   *99*

    Stretch 6: Knee to Chest   *102*

    Stretch 7: Knee Across   *104*

    Stretch 8: Walk to Toes   *106*

8 Designing Your Own Routine   *109*

The Full Shower Routine for Headache,   *111*
Stiff Neck, or Upper Back Pain

The Full Shower Routine for the Middle Back   *113*

The Full Bathtub Routine for the Lower Back   *115*

The Full Hot Tub Routine for the Whole Back   *118*

A Mini-Routine for the Neck and Upper Back   *122*

A Mini-Routine for the Middle Back   *124*

A Mini-Routine for the Lower Back   *126*

A MicroRoutine for the Neck and Upper Back   *129*

A Micro-Routine for the Middle Back   *130*

A Micro-Routine for the Lower Back   *130*

9 Advanced Relaxation Techniques   *131*

Relaxation 1: Progressive Relaxation   *132*

Relaxation 2: Breath-Counting Meditation   *134*

Relaxation 3: Relaxed Muscle Visualization   *136*

Progressive Realization With Visualization: *138*
A Combination

10 Lasting Relief   *139*

Introduction

It is my sincere desire that you will find this book to be informative, helpful, and *useful*. As a chiropractor, I treat people every day who have back pain of one kind or another. My first job is to relieve the pain. My second job is to keep the pain from coming back.

The first job involves tools of my trade such as spinal manipulation and other chiropractic therapies. Since most back problems are "musculoskeletal," I treat the muscles with techniques such as physical therapy (e.g., heat, cold, ultrasound, electrical muscle stimulation) as well as giving attention to the proper alignment of the bones.

Although it is not appropriate, safe, or even possible for patients to manipulate their own bones, I believe that teaching people to manipulate their own soft tissue (muscles), combined with an ongoing exercise program, is the key to keeping the pain from coming back. Self-help — that is, what people do between appointments to help themselves — has as much importance as what I do with them *during* the appointments. This book combines self-help techniques for the back in a new way — utilizing the marvelous qualities of hot water.

— *Dr. Patrick Horay*

As a writer of nearly two dozen instructional methods ranging from music to meditation, I always enjoy taking complicated material and making it simple and useable for readers. But it was a special pleasure working with Dr. Horay on this book, as learning to integrate just a few minutes a day of his *Hot Water Therapy* into my daily life has been great for my own chronically stiff and painful back!

— *David Harp, M.A.*

1

About the Method

Who Needs This Book?

Chances are *you* do, if you picked this book up after noticing the title. And that's no surprise, since an estimated eight out of ten Americans will experience at least one disabling episode of lower back pain in their lives. Even worse, 75 million suffer repeated attacks of back distress, a number increasing by 7 million new victims each year. Many millions more suffer from stiff neck, chronic headaches, and a variety of joint and muscle problems.

A variety of invitations welcome people into this popular but not very exclusive club. Accidents strike responsible citizens and daredevils alike, often exerting a lingering hold on the back long after the recovery process would seem to be over. Sports injuries are common among weekend warriors, who try to coax a week's worth of exercise from a few intensive hours of play and an unprepared, poorly conditioned body.

Stress alone can place a stranglehold on the muscles of the back and neck, especially for those who sit daily in front of a desk or a computer. And even the normal aging process, if not countered by a focused exercise program, leads to increasing stiffness and distress with the years.

It's abundantly clear that there are many opportunities to join the Bad Back Club. Now the question is: What can you do to avoid or cancel your membership?

What's the *Only* Long-Term Remedy for Your "Bad Back"? A Long-Term Exercise Program!

There are many ways of dealing with back, neck, and shoulder problems, but only one offers a good chance of a "permanent" solution. Painkillers and muscle relaxants may help, but they are addictive and a short-term aid at best. Bed rest is boring after a few weeks. Surgery is risky, and chiropractors are expensive when used on an ongoing basis. There is no substitute for a long-term exercise program that gently stretches and strengthens the muscles of the back and neck, whether the problem was originally caused by sports or inactivity, car accident or arthritis. This is true even if the other "remedies," from bed rest to surgery, are utilized.

Doctors, chiropractors, and physical therapists each have their own way to treat back pain. Sometimes the methods overlap, and sometimes they don't. But the one thing on which all agree is that a continuing daily program of stretching and exercise is an essential part of any long-term solution for most victims of back pain. You may wonder who has enough time these days to spend on an ongoing program of physical therapy. The surprise answer is that *you* do. The suggestions described in this book can make those essential exercises and stretches an enjoyable and easily integrated part of your day, every day.

What's So Different About This Method?

There are two main differences between the method of relieving back pain described in this book, and the methods used in any other book that suggest exercise as therapy.

Difference 1: A Physio-therapy Clinic... In Your Bathroom?

Nearly every American home contains two therapeutic devices, which, if used effectively, can alleviate not only upper and lower back pain, but muscle and joint problems of any type. They also offer a pleasing if unorthodox environment for therapy, one that is warmer and more comfortable than any hard floor, and that always offers privacy. The names of these amazing instruments? Your bathtub, and your shower. Some lucky folks may even have a third one — a hot tub!

You see, hydrotherapy, which is a fancy name for doing any kind of exercise in hot water, has been used for years to work with severely disabled or acutely injured patients in hospital settings. But the same methods can be adapted for use in less extreme situations. They can even be used as preventive measures for anyone with back, neck, or shoulder problems.

Doing hydrotherapy at home combines the time-honored effectiveness of exercising in hot water with the convenience of doing something you'd probably do anyway — that is, taking your daily shower or bath. As you are about to learn, hot water can dramatically increase the therapeutic effects of exercise.

Difference 2: The Minimal Time Commitment

Plenty of exercise-based programs promise to help your back. There are yoga programs and weight training programs, calisthenic programs and hang-upside-down-from-your-feet programs. But all of these programs have at least one drawback — they require a considerable daily time commitment. That means that most people, no matter what good intentions they start out with, won't continue doing them for long. And one thing that most experts agree on, no matter which program they prescribe, is that the exercises must be practiced regularly — at least for as long as the patient wants his or her back pain to stay away!

The purpose of this book is to help you to help your back, neck, and shoulders. This simple, usable program encourages you to integrate exercises regularly into your daily schedule, without taking lots of "time out" to do them.

Since some of you have less time to commit to your body than others, the exercises in the coming chapters can be combined into full routines, mini-routines, and micro-routines. Chapter 9 will help you pick the routine that makes the most sense for you, depending on what hurts and your schedule. Even the busiest of folks can spare a few seconds for a ten second micro-routine. Mini-routines take just a few minutes longer, clocking in at two or three minutes. And once you've experienced the benefits of this simple program, you'll probably want to make time for the full routines, which themselves take only ten or fifteen minutes to complete.

Whichever time options fit your lifestyle best, you'll find that doing even a little to help your back on a day-to-day basis is significantly better than deciding to do nothing at all, "because it would take too long." Consistency is the key to significant and lasting improvement.

What's in the Rest of the Book

The next few chapters provide some background information — on hot water, your body, and your pain — that you'll want to know before you begin Hot Water Therapy. The information in Chapter 2 will help you use hot water safely and efficiently; Chapter 3 will help you understand how it works its magic on your body. By Chapter 4 you'll return to thinking about what parts of your body hurt, and when. If you end up philosophizing a little on modern life and the perils thereof, that's okay, too.

Chapters 5, 6, and 7 present the three main steps of this method: deep massage, exercise, and stretching. You'll want to go through these sections carefully, to see which specific massages, exercises, and stretches seem most likely to help you and your back. The general area guides — such as "neck" or "trapezius" — can help you identify the techniques that relate most directly to your trouble spots. Illustrations and step-by-step directions will help you follow each move easily.

Since the best program is one that includes all three steps, Chapter 8 offers instructions for designing a customized Hot Water Therapy program that will fit your own unique body and schedule. You can decide which techniques to use, and how much time you are willing to spend each day on saving your neck and back. This will determine the composition of the full, mini-, and micro-routines that you use.

Chapter 9 presents an advanced step to add to your program: relaxation techniques. Part of the advantage of exercising in hot water is that it makes relaxation relatively simple. Stepping into your tub or shower will automatically begin to relax you, and a few moments of soaking and breathing deeply will prepare you to begin the routines. For those who have the time and dedication, the advanced relaxation techniques can deepen the effectiveness of the hot water routine. Letting go of stress — both in your muscles and your mind — is a crucial component of any therapeutic program, and thus relaxation belongs in every routine that you do.

Finally, in Chapter 10, you'll find helpful hints for avoiding back problems by cultivating good sitting, standing, and working habits. Now that you know what's in store for you, turn the page and start planning for improvement.

A Brief Preview of the
Hot Water Therapy Routines

You'll find all the details in the coming chapters. For now, keep in mind that each section is only part of a comprehensive routine that will include the following:

1. Relaxation in hot water, following the regular cleansing parts of your shower or bath.

2. Deep massage to locate and loosen trouble spots.

3. Gentle, rhythmic exercise to flush muscles and improve circulation.

4. A final stretch to complete flushing of muscles and increase flexibility and tone.

5. Cool down.

6. Return to life with your pain relieved, a stronger back, better back habits, and plans to keep exercising!

2

About Hot Water

The Magic of Hot Water

There is something almost magical about hot water. It was probably in the environment of warm water that the primordial soup coalesced into the dance of spinning molecules known as life. All the conditions had to be just right — plus something extra. Something that calls life out of chaos; something that heals. Slipping into a warm bath, a part of you remembers and allows itself to be supported and buoyed up, warmed and nurtured to the core. It reminds you to let go of mental and physical tension, to give up all the striving and activity, to just be held by the penetrating warmth.

The human race has intuitively recognized the enormous benefits of hot water. Natural hot springs, once discovered, often became sacred areas for regeneration. Many of these developed into centers for healing. As recently as the nineteenth and early twentieth centuries, people flocked to sites of natural hot water — spas — to take "the cure." Hoping to be cured of such diseases as tuberculosis or gout, many certainly experienced some measure of healing. Fortunately, today many of the diseases that people hoped hot water would help have been eradicated through better diet, modern hygiene, clean drinking water, immunization programs, and miracle drugs.

The advent of the modern bathroom has brought hot water into almost every home. It's easy to become accustomed, even blasé, to the ubiquity of hot water, and forget some of its healing benefits. Hot water is more than just a convenience. Used properly, it is a powerful therapeutic tool which you can use in the convenience and privacy of your own bathroom.

What Happens in Hot Water

When you first encounter hot water in the shower, the tub, or the hot tub, it takes your body a few minutes to adjust to the new temperature sensation. During these moments, you experience a temporary increase in blood pressure as the circulatory system responds to the new environment. Blood rushes to the skin, where it is warmed by the hot water. This causes the blood vessels to expand and the blood pressure to drop back down. The rush of warmed blood then penetrates deeper into the tissue below the skin, bringing more oxygen. It also brings a soothing, relaxing sensation as the warmed blood continues to expand more vessels. Even chronically tight muscles, which are responsible for much back pain, begin to relax. That allows the free movement necessary for exercise and stretching.

At the same time that the muscles begin to relax, the nerves are soothed and pain is relieved. As the heat goes deeper, your body temperature may increase to as high as 99°F or more. The rate at which your body uses oxygen and excretes waste material increases, and so does your heart rate and respiration. This is a beneficial effect, helping your body eliminate metabolic waste products. You'll probably begin to sweat, particularly on the face. And you'll begin to feel good all over.

You'll find more about the physiological effects of hot water in the next chapter, About Your Body. For now, scan the lists below to see what Hot Water Therapy offers, and whether it's right for your body.

Physiological Effects of Hot Water

1. Temporarily increased blood pressure followed by decreased blood pressure.
2. Increased superficial circulation.
3. Increased blood supply to muscles.
4. General muscle relaxation, relief of muscle spasm.
5. Increased heart rate.
6. Increased blood volume.
7. Promotion of sweating and increased elimination of metabolic waste.
8. Increased metabolism with more oxygen to the tissue and increasing carbon dioxide production.
9. Increased respiration rate.
10. Stimulation of the immune system and increased anti-body production.
11. Stimulation of liver chemistry and lactic acid conversion.
12. Sedation of sensory motor neurons and pain relief.

Indications for Hot Water Therapy

1. Back pain
2. Arthritis

3. Neuralgia
4. Muscle spasm and muscle tension
5. Sprains and strains
6. Stiffness
7. Bruises and contusions

Contraindications for Hot Water Therapy

Hot water therapy is *not* advised when the following conditions are present. Keep in mind, too, that the technique is *not* appropriate for infants and very young children.

1. Acute fever
2. Severe cardiac complications
3. Seizures
4. Acute bleeding, open wounds, pressure sores
5. Acute skin infections, contagious skin rashes
6. Vascular disease
7. Thermal nerve deficiency
8. Incontinence of bladder/bowel
9. Severe hydrophobia
10. Malignancy or active T.B.

Precautions Regarding Hot Water Therapy

Check with your healthcare professional if you have any of the following conditions, and would like to try hot water therapy.

1. Pregnancy
2. Acute injury
3. Loss of sensation — absent or impaired
4. Postural hypotension

5. Cardiac history

6. Diabetes

7. Obesity or physical disability

8. Impaired balance

How Hot a Bath?

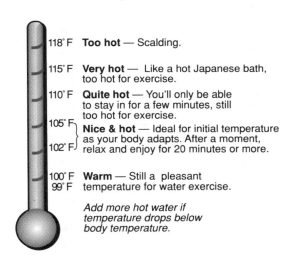

118° F **Too hot** — Scalding.

115° F **Very hot** — Like a hot Japanese bath, too hot for exercise.

110° F **Quite hot** — You'll only be able to stay in for a few minutes, still too hot for exercise.

105° F
Nice & hot — Ideal for initial temperature as your body adapts. After a moment,
102° F relax and enjoy for 20 minutes or more.

100° F **Warm** — Still a pleasant
99° F temperature for water exercise.

Add more hot water if temperature drops below body temperature.

Heat tolerance is one of those individual preferences, so when bathing, find what feels best for you. Don't scald or parboil yourself! Remember that hot water has many physiological effects, and take these into account for therapeutic and safety purposes. For example, hot water lowers blood pressure, so be very careful when beginning to stand up out of a bathtub or hot tub, especially if it is very hot. If you feel at all light-headed or dizzy, proceed with great caution. Sit for a while first, and let your upper body cool down out of the water before attempting to stand up.

For your own convenience, you may want to keep a non-breakable glass of water nearby, along with a damp wash cloth. You sweat a lot in hot water, particularly on your head, so drink some water when you're thirsty and wipe your face with the cool damp wash cloth.

For Additional Luxury...

A nifty way to turn your bath into an herbal bath is to drop a bag of chamomile or mint tea into your bath water. Both will add soothing effects and smell great. They also won't dry the skin as much as soaps, perfumes, and bubble baths.

Shower Safety

Since bathtubs and shower stalls are inherently wet, slippery, and dangerous places to be, a couple of shower safety suggestions are appropriate. Always keep both feet firmly planted on the floor of the shower and bend the knees for extra stability while doing any of the routines suggested. Traction tape on the tub floor surface and strategic grab bars will also be helpful if your particular shower seems at all risky. These investments are well worth the expense to make your bathroom more effective and safe as a therapy setting.

After any of the hot water therapy routines, please take care not to get chilled afterwards. This might undo the benefits you've just worked hard to achieve. The longer the time you've spent doing your routines, the longer the cool down time you should allow. Just keep a towel wrapped around yourself, and enjoy the tapering warmth of the steam in the room.

Two Shower Suggestions

Your health is important, and so is the health of this planet. If you're using your shower for hot water therapy, two suggestions will improve the effectiveness of your shower *and* keep it ecologically sensitive. Choose your favorite.

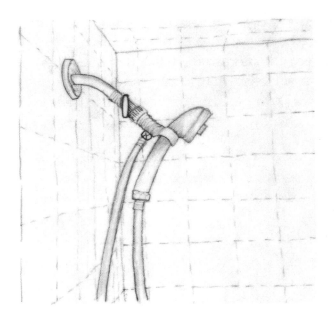

Flow Restrictor

A flow restrictor device can be installed just in front of any shower head. It can be purchased at most plumbing supply or hardware stores. This device will allow you to modulate the flow of water without affecting the temperature. A long shower routine can deplete the water in your hot water heater, causing an abrupt end to your hot water therapy. An empty hot water heater may also adversely affect your popularity with other people in your household, as well as waste water.

A great way to use this flow restrictor device in your shower routine is to take a hand towel into the shower with you. Drape it across your neck and shoulders while the restricted flow of warm water soaks into it. This damp warm towel will prolong the positive effects of hot water while you do your therapy — and will save water at the same time.

New Shower Head

The second suggestion is to purchase a new water-conserving shower head that aerates and focuses the water in a variety of ways. Many also come with an extra length of tubing or hose which allows better handheld placement for localized therapy.

3

About Your Body

Since preparing you for medical school is not the aim of this book, you won't be asked to worry about precisely how the two hundred-odd bones, six hundred-odd muscles, and dozens of joints work to make the human body the engineering marvel that it is. Instead, you'll find enough simplified background information to help you understand the main hows and whys of Hot Water Therapy.

Throughout this section, keep in mind the term "musculoskeletal system." It points to the important interrelation between muscles and bones in your body. While you may feel pain in both places, the muscles are the key point of intervention — for a doctor and for you. In an office, of course, a qualified chiropractor or osteopath can manipulate your bones. But even then, gentle muscle intervention is essential to lasting recovery. Because "soft tissue" such as muscle is relatively simple to manipulate, home therapy becomes possible and effective. That's where most of the techniques described in this book are applied, and where the discussion in this chapter begins. You'll see how various elements work together to cause problems — and to allow a universal solution.

About Your Muscles

It is tempting to think of muscles as rubber bands that can be stretched and released. Actually, muscles work in exactly the opposite way. Unlike rubber bands (which become tighter the longer they are), a muscle is longer when *at rest*, and contracts to become shorter and tighter when in use.

Muscles are attached to bones, and move the bones only by contracting (that is, by making themselves shorter).

This is why muscles are almost always arranged in pairs — so that one can contract while the other relaxes, in order to move a bone. Your bicep and tricep work together to bend your arm, for instance. When you raise your hand to "make a muscle," the muscle tissue of your bicep shortens, while your tricep muscle remains relaxed and long.

How Muscles Work

Muscle tissue is made up of a multitude of tiny fibers, shaped like threads. The fibers of a large muscle can be over a foot long, and the fibers of a small one much shorter than an inch. It is the contractile action of these fibers that causes a muscle to shorten, and thus move the bone to which the muscle is attached. Veins, arteries, and nerves are also found within muscles.

When you want to tense or tighten a muscle, your brain sends signals along your nerves to the desired muscle, and the fibers of that muscle contract among themselves, shortening the length of the muscle.

Unfortunately, muscular tension is not always under your conscious control. When you are driving, typing, or viewing a computer screen for hours on end, the muscles of your back, neck, and shoulders may tend to tighten up, even if you don't consciously will or even want them to. And many people react to stress of almost any sort by habitually contracting their neck and shoulder muscles. What's so bad about that? You'll see!

Muscles and Blood

One of the most basic needs of all living tissue, including muscle tissue, is an adequate blood supply. Blood carries oxygen and other nutrients into the muscle via the arteries, and removes waste products such as carbon dioxide and lactic acid via the veins. Since these blood vessels run through the muscle itself, the state of the muscle tissue — either relaxed, contracted, or an alternating combination of the two as the muscle is used — has a powerful effect on the circulation of the blood.

When a muscle is in a relaxed condition, its muscle fibers are spaced relatively far apart. There is plenty of room for blood to circulate amongst the cells of the fibers, bringing in nourishment and carrying away waste products.

As a muscle is used in a rhythmic way, such as walking, running, swimming, gathering berries, or any of the other common human activities that have been practiced since prehistory, the alternating contractions and relaxations of the muscle fiber actually help to send the blood back to the heart. This keeps the muscle soft, pliable, and supple.

When contracted, the muscle fibers are more densely spaced, leaving less room for blood to circulate. Veins and arteries, as well as nerves, are constricted, just as the flow of water through a garden hose is choked if you squeeze it tightly with your hand. Less oxygen and nutrients enter the muscle tissue, and waste products accumulate as less can be carried away by the decreased blood flow. This may surprise you, since a contracted muscle is working harder than a relaxed one, and actually needs *more* nutrients and produces *more* waste products just when the blood flow slows down.

Sound discouraging? It needn't be. In normal use, muscles alternate contraction with relaxation. When contraction is held and tension builds up, the massage, gentle exercise, and stretching techniques of Hot Water Therapy can relax the muscles and increase blood flow, flushing waste products and bringing nutrients to the muscles.

The Dangers of Chronic Muscle Tension

As you may have guessed from the above description of a muscle in contraction, this is a normal condition, but it isn't a healthy one to sustain very long.

Maintaining even a partial state of contraction over a long period of time — as when you work, drive, or worry — can have numerous negative effects. The buildup of waste products, especially lactic acid, can cause pain and a tendency to cramp. An average desk worker may have as much tension in his neck and shoulders after a long day as a marathon runner has in her legs after a long race — and as much lactic acid. The difference is that the runner probably has better toned muscles, as well as a routine for relieving tension.

An even more serious problem is that a chronic state of contraction can make the muscle fibers permanently shorten, reducing the range of motion that is possible without tearing the muscle fiber. This, naturally, leads to torn muscles, even for those who don't fall victim to the "weekend warrior" syndrome. Even minor accidents or overusage can tear short, tight muscles.

When the fibers of a muscle have been torn, which is typically what happens when you suffer a "strain," they do not always grow back as normal fiber. Instead, they can be replaced by scar tissue, which does not relax and contract as does normal muscle fiber. Scar tissue tends to constrict nerves and blood vessels even after the injury has been "fully healed." Thus people who have torn muscles in accidents, for instance, are often vulnerable to repeated injury in the same place.

The Splinting Reflex

It seems unfair, but once a muscle becomes tight, its tendency is not to relax, but to become even tighter. This is due to what physiologists refer to as the "splinting reflex."

When a muscle is injured or in pain for any reason, the splinting reflex acts to stiffen the muscle and prevent it from moving. This works well in the case of accidental injury. In the good old days, if you fell down and sprained your ankle while hunting mastodons far from the cave. The natural splinting reflex would stiffen your leg enough to hobble home.

Now, however, muscular pain, rather than being due to injury, is likely to be caused by shortening of the back muscles due to chronic tension. When the splinting reflex kicks in, the muscle tightens even further, clamping down on its blood vessels and nerves, and the pain increases. The greater the pain, the tighter the muscle clamps down. The tighter it gets, the more you hurt. You can't win, and may eventually end up with your back in spasm. Unless, of course, you intervene to relax and lengthen the muscles with a technique like Hot Water Therapy!

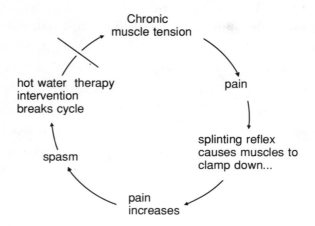

Chronic
muscle tension

hot water therapy
intervention
breaks cycle

pain

splinting reflex
causes muscles to
clamp down...

spasm

pain
increases

Breaking the Cycle of Pain and Tension

Muscles and Nerves

Chronically contracted muscles can also tend to pinch or constrict the nerves that run through them. Some authorities believe that this is one of the major causes of the common but hard-to-diagnose aches and pains of increasing age.

You don't need to be a senior citizen to suffer from this type of discomfort. Sometimes a muscle will develop a hard, sensitive spot within it that may range from the size of a large pinhead to that of a thumbnail. This happens most often with muscles that suffer from chronic tension.

It appears that these knotty spots, in addition to being painful themselves, can cause what is called "referred pain" in unrelated parts of the body. When this happens, the sensitive spot is often called a "trigger point." A classic case of this is the tension headache, when tightly knotted trigger points in the back or neck refer pain to the head. Fortunately, when these trigger points are located, massaged, exercised, and stretched, the headache will often diminish as well. Although it seems paradoxical, direct massage pressure to relax the tissue and flush the blood from the painful spot may in many cases relax or even repair damage in the entire muscle.

No one knows why this works. A number of alternative medical disciplines, including acupuncture, rolfing, and trigger point injection therapy offer theories on the subject. Regardless of the reason, direct massage of sensitive muscular spots can often be part of an effective way of working with back and neck pain. Deep massage techniques are an important part of Hot Water Therapy, and will be discussed in detail in Chapter 5.

About Your Bones

Bones are the other main component of the musculoskeletal system. A broken arm bone or genetically misshapen thigh bone will impair the ability of even the most powerful and flexible muscles to function. However, with such extreme situations excepted, the bones themselves are rarely the original cause of back or muscle pain. More often, the problems lie with the way injured or chronically contracted muscles exert pressure on the bones to which they are attached.

Bones are connected to muscles by strands of tissue called tendons. When muscles are chronically tight, the points at which the tendon attaches to both the muscle and the bone carry extra stress. This often causes pain, even if the muscle fiber has not been torn.

Even pain and difficulties with the twenty-four tiny, movable vertebrae that form the spine are most often caused by muscular problems which force the vertebrae out of proper alignment. And while the chiropractor's skilled hands can often adjust the vertebrae back into shape, if the underlying muscles are not in good condition, the spine will soon twist back into its contorted configuration. The doctor may be able to get your bones into their proper places, but it's you and your muscles that have to keep them there!

Joints

Joints are the parts of the body that allow bones to remain connected to each other without touching. There are many different types of joints (the shoulder is clearly quite different from the hip, and the elbow from the ankle), but most share certain common features.

In most joints, the parts of the bones that are nearly but not quite touching are covered with a bone-like but softer tissue called cartilage. The entire joint is surrounded by a tough layer of tissue called the joint capsule, which keeps the entire area bathed in fluid.

When *gently* stimulated by movement, cells within the joint capsule produce fluid, but when "jammed" or jarred by violent motion these cells can become inflamed. In this case, they oversecrete their lubricating fluid, causing additional pain and swelling.

After injury to the area of a joint, scar tissue sometimes replaces the fluid-producing membrane. In this case, the tissue then stops secreting fluid, and the joint becomes excessively dry. This too causes pain.

The buoyancy provided by warm water in a bath or hot tub will decrease the pressure of gravity on a weak or injured joint, allowing the joint to be stimulated more gently and with less pain. This can be particularly helpful for people with arthritis.

4

Where Does It Hurt?

It's probably not too much of an exaggeration to say that there are two kinds of people: people who have "bad backs," and people who don't have bad backs...yet. If you're reading this book, you probably fall into the former category.

What to Do First

Whether your problem is new or old, periodic or chronic, there are two things that you must do. First, a professional medical opinion must be sought, from doctor, chiropractor, or osteopath. While extremely uncommon, back pain can sometimes be a symptom of serious diseases as diverse as bone tumors, prostate cancer, or bowel obstruction. All of these must be ruled out by competent diagnosis before treatment can begin, and this is the responsibility of a professional. A professional can also guide you through the acute phase of injuries such as whiplash or torn muscles from a weekend soccer game, when rest may be more appropriate than exercise.

Second, when the treatment and healing period prescribed by your caregiver is over, you need to begin an exercise program to condition the muscles of your back or neck to avoid a recurrence of the problem. Remember: once the back or neck has been injured, it will be more prone to re-injury. This makes a preventive maintenance program even more essential!

The worse the shape your muscles, bones, and joints are in, the gentler and more gradual the exercise program must be. But no one's body is in such bad shape that it cannot be helped by the proper hot water routine.

No matter what particular form your back problems take, you're really the only person who can decide and know exactly what you need to work on, and know how much time and energy you can spare to do it. A doctor, chiropractor, or osteopath can help, but real progress can only be made if you take responsibility for ongoing soft tissue work in between appointments. Becoming aware of the specific nature of your problem is a good place to begin.

Where Do You Hurt?

For some people, the answer to this question is obvious. Painfully obvious. For others, having a "bad back" or a "stiff neck" may be as far as they've wanted to think about it.

Now is a good time to focus your attention on your body and pinpoint areas of pain or tightness. Everyone's body is different. But all human beings suffer from the same general structural problem: backs take the brunt of upright use. Most modern human beings share two other problems: too much sitting, and not enough varied exercise. Thus people tend to share common trouble spots, as well. Five general categories of "ache area" will be used to distinguish the exercises and stretches on the following pages: *neck, trapezius, upper back, mid-back,* and *lower back.*

Often one muscle's tightness will cause neighboring problems as well, and "referred pain" can make it difficult to tell exactly where the pain originates. Fortunately, many of the exercises in the Hot Water Therapy program will have a beneficial effect on an entire area. It helps to locate the primary source of pain, but knowing a general target area will help you, too.

What's Going On Under There?

Instead of worrying about the Latin names of muscles, it's more productive to think about where it hurts. That's why this book's division of exercise area is based more on the problematic region of the body than the underlying musculature. For your educational enjoyment, though, you might examine the illustrations below to locate specific muscles responsible for much back trouble. Remember that these muscles overlap, the *trapezius* stretching across much of the upper and middle back, and the *rhomboids* and the *levitor scapulae* working just underneath. The following sections will help you see what each muscle does more clearly.

You'll also want to examine the illustration of common pressure points and referred pain areas. A pressure point is any tender, knotty area that hurts if you press into it. Over time and extended use, or following a trauma, a pressure point can develop into a trigger point, radiating pain to other areas of your back and body. Ideally, you'll intervene *before* this happens with gentle massage, exercise and stretching. You'll find more about pressure points in the chapter on Deep Massage. For now, look at the illustration that follows — and think about where *your* pain starts. The illustration indicates common pressure points with bull's-eyes, and areas where pain might tend to radiate over time with arrows. All points can develop on either side of the back — and you might develop unique points of your own!

And remember, *everything* in your back, from the head down, is hitched to everything else — so it will be worth your while to at least experiment with *all* of the suggested techniques.

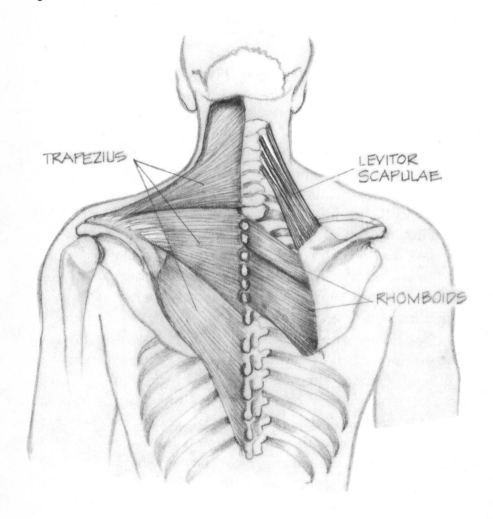

Three Major Back Muscle Groups

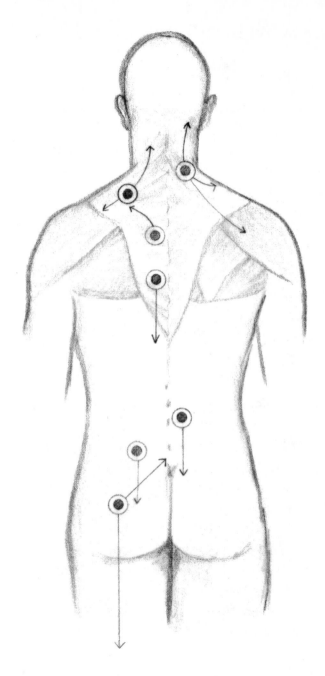

**Common Pressure Points
with Possible Pain Radiation**

The Most Common Trouble Areas

The Neck

Pain and stiffness in the neck is usually rooted in the interaction between the seven vertebrae of the neck (called the cervical vertebra) and the muscles that move those vertebrae. These problem muscles tend to be the ones that run down the back of the neck from the base of the skull, and include the *levitor scapulae*, which raise and lower the shoulder blades, among other things, and the *trapezius*, which will be discussed separately.

Tension headaches are often related to tension in the neck, so if this is a problem for you, the neck routines are a "must do."

The Shoulders

When people complain of shoulder pain, they may be referring either to a problem with the musculature or joint that connects the arm to the shoulder, or to pain in the uppermost extreme left and uppermost extreme right parts of the back next to the actual shoulder area.

Problems with the "joint" part of the shoulder (called "rotator cuff" injury) must often be dealt with by surgery or micro-surgery, and are beyond the scope of this book. But for those of you whose pain lies near but not in the shoulder joint, two hot water routines are suggested — one for the trapezius muscles, and one for the muscles of the upper back. If you are not sure which of these two areas will help you most, try both and see.

The Trapezius Muscles

Most people think that these are the small triangular muscles on each side of the lower neck, covering an area roughly the size and shape of a coat hanger. And, indeed, this is the area that will be focused on in the exercises for the trapezius. Yet, like an iceberg, a large portion of the trapezius musculature is out of sight and mind, extending down nearly to the lower back.

The trapezius is a versatile trouble spot. Tension in these muscles can cause headaches and pain running up the neck, as well as upper and middle back pain. Particularly troublesome and prevalent is pain occurring at the edge of the shoulder blade closest to the spine. The upper trapezius also has the distinction of hosting the single most common pressure or trigger point found in the human body (and a very painful one it is).

The Upper Back

The upper back is the area from the shoulder blades up into the neck.

Much upper back pain is due to trapezius tension, but other muscle groups can contribute to discomfort in this area, including the rhomboids, which run between the shoulder blades and the spine on each side. Tightness in the rhomboids, as in the trapezius muscles, can cause persistent pain between the edge of the shoulder blade and the spine. Many computer operators and other varieties of desk workers know firsthand just how unpleasant this can be.

The Middle Back

The middle back area extends from the top to the bottom of your rib cage.

Tightness in the lower portions of the trapezius muscles can cause pain in the middle back, as can tension in the long, thin muscles that run from the base of the skull to the pelvis (not pictured). Referred pain from trigger points or tension in these muscles can sometimes be felt in the buttocks , in which case it is often called by the old-fashioned name of lumbago.

The Lower Back

The lower back describes the area from the bottom of your rib cage down into your buttocks.

Most lower back pain occurs in the region where the five lumbar vertebrae of the lower back join the solid bone of the sacrum (not pictured). Interestingly enough, many of the muscles that can help this part of the body remain pain-free are not back muscles at all, but abdominal muscles. Thus, exercises for this area are aimed at strengthening the stomach musculature as well as relaxing that of the back.

The Tight Shoulders, Flabby Tummy Syndrome

For many people, tight muscles in the upper and lower back interact with weak stomach muscles to create a "double whammy" problem. Tight shoulders jam joints in the area, and alter the normal curve of the neck. Flabby tummies make muscles in the lower back work without balance or support. This makes the lower back a prime candidate for the pain/ tightness cycle of the "splinting reflex," which often escalates into the dreaded and incapacitating "back spasm." The solution: drop those shoulders, tighten that tummy!

The Entire Back

Some of the exercises and stretches are beneficial for the entire back. So, no matter what specific trouble spots you may have, try to work these into your routine.

When Do You Hurt?

Unless your back is very bad, you probably don't hurt all of the time. And even if you do, you probably hurt more at certain times than others. Now might be a good time to focus your mental attention on your body, and try to recall when you hurt and in what specific places. Is it while you're doing something in particular, or right after? When you've talked on the phone for a long time? Lifted something? Driven a distance? Sat all day? If nothing comes to mind right away, keep the question "When does my back hurt?" or "When does it hurt worse than usual?" in the "back" of your mind (so to speak).

Weekly Pain Log

An efficient way to discover what makes you hurt is to keep a pain log. This can be as simple as learning to jot down a note in your calendar or day book whenever you experience back tension or pain. Try to include where you were or what you were doing before or during the pain. After a few days or weeks, you will likely see some patterns emerging.

The Pain Log
(Make several copies)

Day and Time	Trouble Area	Radiation (i.e., up neck into head)	Character (sharp, shooting, or dull ache)

The Pain Log
(continued)

Intensity (1-mild discomfort to 5-extreme pain)	Activities (i.e., phone, desk-work, driving, gardening)	Stress Level (1-at ease to 5-over-whelmed)	Coping Strategy (i.e., aspirin, rubbing, Hot Water Therapy)	Effect of Coping Strategy

If you like, keep a more accurate record using the printed chart. There is room for you to write a few times each day for a week. Make a habit of stopping briefly at convenient breaks such as meal times to reflect on the state of your back, and on your activities, for the preceding few hours. Describe the nature and intensity of the pain as clearly as you can. Indicate exactly where it hurts, and where it radiates. This information can be of great use to your doctor, osteopath, or chiropractor. Ideally, it will help you to reduce or eliminate back pain by enabling you to avoid its causes, or at least know when to take extra care of yourself. And a great way to do that is by intensifying your use of Hot Water Therapy!

Before you begin to fill out your Weekly Pain Log, be sure to make several blank copies. When you turn to a new one, be sure to save the old ones. You may want to compile them in a notebook or a folder.

If Bad Backs Are the Symptom, What's the Disease?

Perhaps the problem is not so much the literal pain-in-the-neck at the top of the shoulders, but the more figurative pain-in-the-neck of a hectic and harried lifestyle. Think of the stereotyped image of a truckdriver, construction worker, or longshoreman afflicted by back pain, and you'll only have part of the picture. The two largest causes of back and neck problems today are mental stress and deskwork.

Mental stress can make you tighten your neck and upper back muscles, as though getting ready to ward off a blow from above. Shoulders come up, neck pulls down, and presto: the human turtle! After a while, it's hard to even recognize the unnaturalness of this position. Shoulders are chronically raised, the possible range of motion of the head is reduced, and the human turtle becomes (to mix an animal metaphor) a sitting duck for the sneeze, slip, or bend that "throws out" an upper back, lower back, or neck.

For those who sit and stare at a desktop or computer screen all day, upper bodies become overdeveloped. This doesn't refer to huge muscles, but to muscles remaining in a state of chronic tension. Simultaneously, lower bodies, and especially abdominal muscles, become weak from disuse, setting the scene for the pain/tightness "splinting cycle" that throws the lower back into agonizing spasm.

If you can learn to understand your bodily discomforts as symptoms of a lifestyle that is dysfunctional in certain ways, you can actually use your back and neck pain to motivate you to change for the better, both physically and mentally. This book, if you use it diligently, will help you to do just that. The last chapter in particular offers some ideas for improving your daily back habits.

Are you ready to begin? The next chapter will start you on your way to building your own complete routines. Deep massage is an essential first step.

5

Deep Massage Techniques

Why Deep Massage Works

Deep massage is just a fancy name for self-massage that concentrates on finding and massaging pressure points, or trigger points. As discussed in the section on muscles and nerves, these tender spots can have a strong effect on the muscles in which they reside, as well as on more distant parts of the body in the form of referred pain.

Even without working on pressure or trigger points, massage can help stimulate the circulation of blood in tense muscles. Massage will also physically loosen the chronically contracted muscle fibers, helping the muscle to reach a more lengthened and relaxed state. For all these reasons, it is an important early step in your routines.

Just a few seconds of deep massage will enhance the effects of the exercises and stretches, so don't neglect this part of the routine even if you are only doing a mini- or a micro-routine. The massage techniques remain the same, whether you do them in the shower, bath, or hot tub. While hot water enhances the healing benefits of these massages, some will even be helpful if you try them "dry" — or with the aid of a hot pack, which you'll learn how to make in a later chapter.

Deep Massage Techniques

Almost any way that you can touch your body should feel good, but here are a few suggestions for those who are not used to self-massage. Please feel free to experiment, and to touch yourself in any way that pleases you. Remember that you may feel occasional tenderness as you work tense muscles; but don't cross the line into pain.

First, as you stand under the shower or soak in the tub, *relax*. A few advanced relaxation techniques will be provided in Chapter 10, but the simple breathing exercise on the next page is a fine way to begin. It will help you get the most of the one to two minutes of deep breathing recommended before any hot water routine, and prepare your body for the benefits to follow.

Second, you'll be introduced to two standard techniques for finding and loosening those tender, knotty pressure points: the finger walk, and the finger stroke. Once you practice these techniques, you'll be able to combine them with specific massage routines.

Finally, you'll be ready to start on the massages themselves. Included here is one for the upper back (including neck and shoulders); one for the lower back; and one for the middle back. Since the middle back is hard to reach, there are instructions for making a handy device to apply pressure to that important middle area. You'll find directions for each massage in a box, along with an illustration of a person demonstrating the movement.

A Touch of Relaxation

While standing, place one hand over your chest, and the other on your stomach. Pretend that your hands are glued to your body. Begin to inhale, pulling out on the hand over your stomach, so that your stomach expands as it fills with air first. When your stomach feels full, do the same with your chest.

When your chest is full of air also, begin to exhale while gently pushing in on your chest, so that the air leaves the chest first. Then gently push in on the stomach, until that area too feels completely empty of air. Repeat the entire process, concentrating on filling the stomach, then the chest, then emptying the chest, and finally the stomach.

Repeat for about ten full breaths, feeling oxygen and steam from the hot water fill you up, as tension and worry melt away.

The Finger Walk:
Searching for Pressure Points

The finger walk is a convenient and natural way to find centers of tension, and apply helpful pressure. Use your fore and middle fingers so that the very tips walk in tiny steps across the muscle. Feel for tender spots that indicate pressure points by gently pressing into the tissue. Don't press so hard that it hurts wherever the fingers walk, but don't just skim over the skin, either. Your fingers should sink into the muscle beneath the skin at least a quarter of an inch.

When you feel a spot that is clearly more tender than the surrounding area, gently press into that spot. Make it hurt slightly. Continue to press with the same degree of pressure until you feel the pain diminish. Generally, this will take from 10 to 30 seconds. When the pain fades, do not press harder. Just let the pain fade out as much as it will, then continue your finger walk, and seek additional tender spots. (See the illustration in Chapter 4 of common pressure points if you have trouble locating your own.)

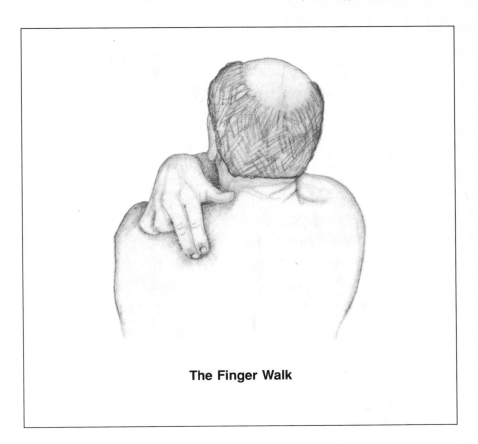

The Finger Walk

The Finger Stroke:
Flushing the Muscle

This stroke helps to increase circulation and flush tightened muscle fiber. For the finger stroke, use the flats of your fingers, as if you're brushing off dust. The difference is that you're pressing more deeply into the muscle. Brush your hand slowly along the length of the muscle, working along the muscle in the direction of your heart. As you work, visualize your hand flushing the muscle to loosen it and increase circulation.

As in the finger walk, try to locate centers of the pain or tightness in the muscle, and press gently into those points when you find them. Rub your fingers in circles around the painful points, too, pressing gently into the tissue and flushing the area. The finger stroke allows broader contact with the hurting muscle than the finger walk, but the idea is the same. If you're not certain just how to do this, don't worry. Just stroke it the way that feels best.

Use enough pressure to depress the tissue, and always begin your stroke further away from the center of the body, and end your stroke closer to the center of the body. You always want to stroke in the direction of the heart.

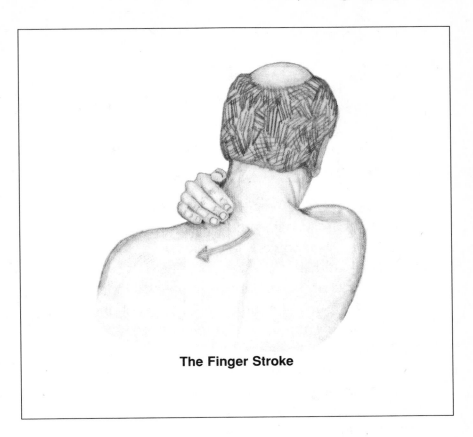

The Finger Stroke

Massage 1:
The Trapezius Walk

shower, bath,　　　　　　*neck, trapezius,*
or hot tub　　　　　　　*upper back*

This deep massage technique should be part of any routine for neck pain, upper back pain, or tension headaches. Reach your left hand up to the base of your skull, and start walking your fingers down along the left side of the center of your neck (not on the spine itself, but just near it) until you reach the base of your neck. Then switch hands and work your way down the shoulder, along the trapezius to the bony area at the top of your left shoulder. Stop and concentrate on any tender spots by pressing into them gently until the pain recedes. Then repeat on the right side, beginning with your right hand at the top of your spine and switching to your left hand as you reach the right trapezius muscle. Work down a little into the upper back, as well.

This is prime real estate for pressure and trigger points. Let your fingers walk carefully, taking tiny steps, so as not to miss any. The illustration in Chapter 4 shows their most common locations, but you'll know 'em if you find 'em — they hurt!

If you make a BackuPressure device as described described in the following pages, you will be able to continue your "walk" down into your middle back, which provides more good territory for pressure points.

The *sacrum* is a triangular bone at the base of the spine, composed of vertebrae that are fused together. Movable, un-fused vertebrae (called the *lumbar vertebrae*) sit on top of the sacrum. That's the problem: moveable parts are attached to the top of a solid base, making the region where the pelvis joins the spine a hotspot for lower back pain. A moment of massage before the lower back exercises and stretches will help circulation in the area, and feel good, too.

Massage 2:
The Sacrum Stroke

shower, bath,   *lower back*
or hot tub

Place your palms on either side of the top of your pelvis, so that you can conveniently use your thumbs to make small circles on the muscles on either side of the spine.

Then work your way down onto the flat, bony part of the back of the pelvis. As you get lower, you may want to reverse your hands and use your fingers instead of your thumbs. Once again, if you find any pressure points, press gently into them until the pain recedes.

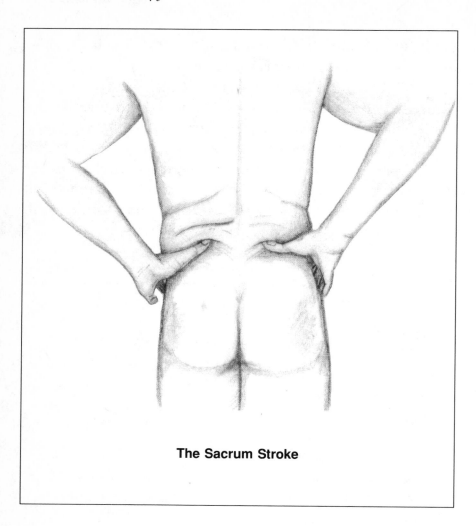

The Sacrum Stroke

How To Make and Use a BackuPressure Device

It's pretty easy to reach the upper and lower parts of your back with your hands, and nearly impossible to reach the middle. So here's a way to make a simple deep pressure device that will let you work with tight muscles and trigger points in this hard-to-reach region.

You'll need:

- Two tennis balls, or balls of similar size and hardness
- Two sturdy rubber bands
- A towel at least 30" long or, even better, an old pair of pantyhose

Place the balls in the center of the towel, next to each other, aligned with the long way of the towel. Or cut one leg from the pantyhose, and slide the balls into the knee area, aligned lengthwise. Roll the towel tightly to form a long tube with the balls in the middle. Pantyhose won't need to be rolled any tighter.

Put the rubber bands around the towel tube or pantyhose leg to hold the balls in place.

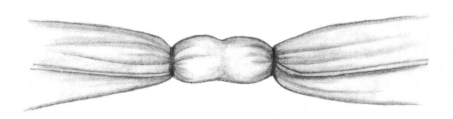

BackuPressure Device

Massage 3: Using
Your BackuPressure Device

shower, bath,   *middle back*
or hot tub

Hold the device by the ends. Position the balls any-where you like on your back, and then lean gently into them. If you do this against a wall, your own weight helps create pressure against the tennis balls. You can use the device to locate pressure points throughout your back. Some people like the firmer pressure of the device even better than the gentler pressure of the fingers. Don't overdo it, though — if you are using the device on a pressure point and the pain doesn't seem to be decreasing after twenty or thirty seconds, back off. You should never feel bruised or hurt after using the device.

When looking for pressure points in the middle back, position the balls on either side of your spine a few inches above your pelvis, and slowly work your way up the back. Lean into the device against the wall or tub side, and probe for tender areas. When you find a point, hold the pressure for 30 to 60 seconds until the tenderness fades.

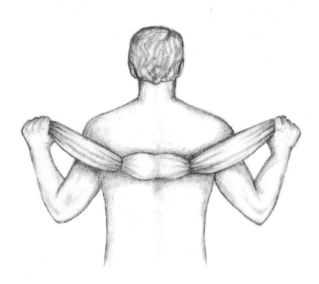

Using the BackuPressure Device on Middle Back

Always move toward your heart, or the center of your body, as you probe. After working up to the middle back from your pelvis, switch up to your shoulders and work down if you want to reach higher regions.

You may find that holding the ends of the device diagonally (with one hand lower, and the other higher) feels better than having both hands at the same level. You can even experiment with holding the device vertically, by having one hand behind your head, and the other behind your lower back.

6

Exercise Techniques

Why Exercise Works

Gentle, rhythmic exercising can help your back and neck in two ways. It will loosen joints and muscles (especially in conjunction with warm water), and it will increase the range of motion that is possible. Certain exercises can do this by contracting and relaxing the muscle fibers that have "gotten used to" being permanently shortened.

Exercise also helps flush muscle tissue that suffers from a permanent state of semi-contraction and decreased blood circulation. As the muscle contracts fully, the blood is pushed out, flushing out toxic materials. As the muscle relaxes, the blood rushes back in, bringing in fresh oxygen and nutrients.

It's a bit like cleaning out a dry, dirty sponge. You wet it, then squeeze it, then wet and squeeze again until the dirty water has been replaced with clear water.

About the Exercises

Some of these exercises are tailored to the shower, while others are specific to the bathtub or hot tub. This will be noted in the upper left corner of the box. The exercises are grouped by appropriate trouble spot, which will be indicated in the upper right of the box. In Chapter 8, you'll learn how to integrate them with massage and stretching into longer and shorter routines for bath, shower, and hot tub usage.

Many of the exercises, particularly those designed for the shower, can be done on dry land as well. These can be useful throughout your day, when you have a free moment but are far from a shower or a bath. Remember, however, that hot water significantly increases the therapeutic effect of these movements by relaxing your body and increasing blood circulation. And caution: high heels or unstable shoes of any sort should be removed before doing any of the dry land standing exercises or stretches!

Whenever possible, in water or not, precede these exercises with at least a few seconds of deep massage directed toward the appropriate muscle group. Most of the exercises are described in sets of six repetitions each. If this seems too many or too few, feel free to adjust the number to suit your own needs.

When exercising in the bath or hot tub, you may want a cushion to soften the hard floor of the tub. A large bath towel is perfect for this purpose, and don't worry about getting it wet. That's what it's made for!

And finally, none of these exercises is supposed to hurt. Pain tells you that you're doing too much; it means a muscle is constricting, when your goal is to stretch and loosen it. Although some tenderness may be involved in initially moving stiff, sore muscles, this feeling should diminish as you continue. If it doesn't, *stop* — before you cross the line into pain. If every possible movement causes pain, you'll need to consult a professional. Also, if you are in the acute phase of an illness or injury, rest or ice may be more appropriate than movement. Review the contraindications for Hot Water Therapy in Chapter 2, and check with a health care professional if you have any doubts.

Exercise 1: Shoulder Lifts.

shower   *neck, trapezius,
                                       upper back*

• Stand comfortably, with your feet about 18 inches apart.

• Imagine that a string runs from the very top of your head to a hook directly above you, so that you are standing as straight and tall as possible. Your spine is extended, and your chin points straight ahead. Perhaps you'd like to visualize your vertebrae as a strand of pearls, dangling loosely on a silken thread held from above. Your shoulders are loose and low, with your arms hanging comfortably at your sides.

• This is the posture you'll want to maintain during all the standing exercises.

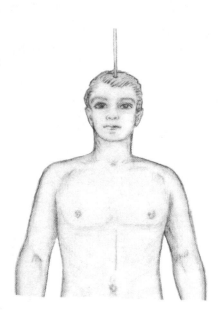

"Hanging from a String" Posture

• Bring your shoulders straight up (not allowing them to move towards the front or the back), as though you were trying to touch them to your ears, but...

• Do not crunch your neck or head at all! Remember that you are "hanging from a string." That means keeping your head and neck completely extended. IMPORTANT: It is better to raise your shoulders less, than to raise them more by "crunching" or "turtling" your neck. Keep your neck elongated.

• Hold the raised position for six seconds, noticing (and relaxing) any tendency to contract the neck or lower the head. Don't forget to breathe!

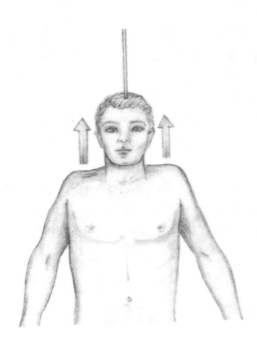

Shoulder Lifts

• Relax the shoulders, and let them settle back in slow motion to a normal position, loose and low. Visualize your shoulders and arms as parts of a very heavy coat, hanging loosely from a coat hanger.

• If you like, use your fingertips to "walk down the sides of your legs" to lower the shoulders as much as possible.

• Repeat the entire process five more times, for a total of six repetitions.

•   Good, erect, posture is an important part of this exercise. So, once again, avoid any tendency to crunch or turtle the neck or lower the head — you are still hanging from that string. Feel your spine straighten and elongate. Feel your arms hanging low, without tension.

When you feel comfortable doing this exercise in a standing position, with no hint of turtling, try it while sitting down in the tub, or even at your desk. Even seated, remember that string from which your head and body are hanging!

Exercise 2: Shoulder Circles

shower   *neck, trapezius,*
                                          upper back

•   This exercise is similar to shoulder lifts, except that instead of simply lifting your shoulders, you will be making circles with them. Begin the same way as in Exercise 1, with your feet comfortably apart, and standing as straight and tall as possible; be sure not to crunch or turtle your neck or head. Your arms and shoulders are hanging loose and low.

•   Without tensing your arms, or moving your torso or head, bring your shoulders as far forward as they can go without beginning to lift up.

•   When your shoulders are as far forward as they can go without lifting, raise them as high as you can without tightening your arms or neck.

•   When they are as high as they can go without turtling the neck or tightening any muscles other than the shoulders, bring them straight back as far as you can get them. Let your elbows bend naturally if they want to.

•   Now drop them as far down as they can go (still in the far back position). Once dropped, bring them to the low and completely relaxed position in which they started.

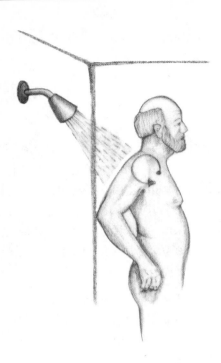

Forward Circle, Almost Completed

• You have now completed one 360 degree shoulder circle. Do it again, trying to maintain one smooth, slow, circular motion rather than four separate jerky motion. Take up to 20 or 30 seconds to complete one circle, at first. Keep your breathing deep and regular, coordinating it with your counting if you like.

• Now do a circle in the other direction. Begin in the low, relaxed shoulder position, move your shoulders back, then up, then forward, then down to complete the circle.

• Repeat the backward circle again in a smooth motion, allowing 20 to 30 seconds for the entire circle.

• Once you're used to the motion, allow six seconds per circle. Repeat three times forward and three backward. Always stretch as far in each direction as you can, without pain.

As with Exercise 1, be careful to avoid any neck tension or turtling during this exercise. Maintain an erect, "hook-hanging" position. When you feel comfortable with the standing version of the exercise, try it sitting, but keep your posture erect.

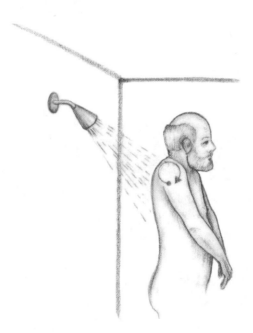

Backward Circle, Almost Completed

Exercise 3: Head Rock

shower   *neck*

• Stand comfortably in the "hanging from a string" posture. Turn your head gently to the left, as far as it will go without pain. Keep your shoulders relaxed, and as low as possible.

• Now, still turned to the left, gently lift your chin as high as it will go *without pain*, eyes on the ceiling. Take three or four seconds to raise it.

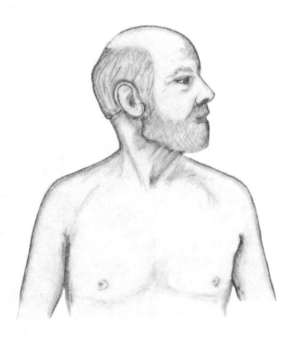

Head Rock, Left Neutral

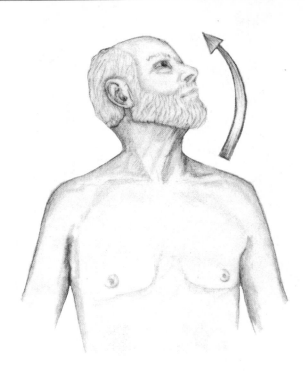

Head Rock, Chin Up

• Gently lower your chin until it's level with your shoulder, still turned to the left. Now keep lowering your chin, with your eyes on the floor, as far as it will go *without pain*. Take three or four seconds to complete.

• If it seems hard to raise or lower your head while it is turned all the way to the left, try turning it less before attempting to raise and lower it.

• Gently lift your chin and return to neutral.

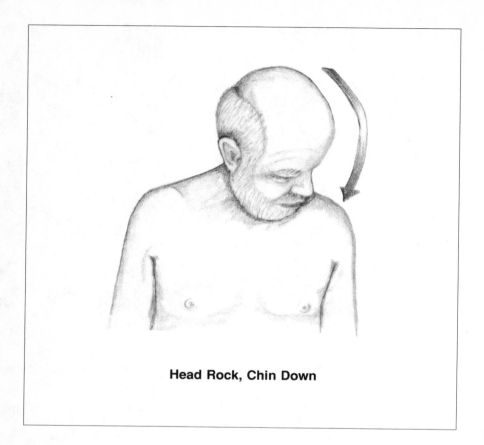

Head Rock, Chin Down

• Repeat five more times to the left for a total of six repetitions, keeping your breathing regular. Then turn to face forward, eyes focused straight ahead.

• Now do the same to the right side, six times. Turn right, chin up, lower to neutral, chin down, back to neutral, repeat. Count about six seconds for the rock up, and six for the rock down, moving smoothly.

If you notice yourself wanting to turtle your neck in order to raise your head, don't! You are better off making less of an up and down movement, and not crunching your neck, then maximizing the up and down by crunching.

Once you can do this one without turtling, practice it while seated.

This exercise may help you become aware of how easy it is to turtle, without even thinking about it. Keep your shoulders low and your neck extended throughout the exercise. Many people turtle when they concentrate on something; try to become aware of this tendency.

Exercise 4: Elbow Across Chest

shower   *middle back*

•   Stand comfortably, in the erect "hanging from a string" position. Your shoulders are low, and your arms comfortably dangling.

•   Touch the fingers of your left hand to your left shoulder, and lift your arm until your left elbow points straight out from your body at shoulder level.

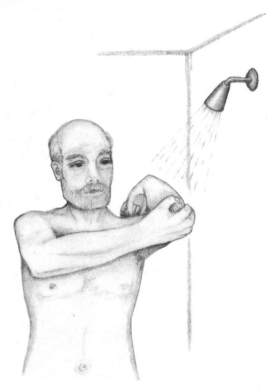

Elbow Across Chest, Left Neutral

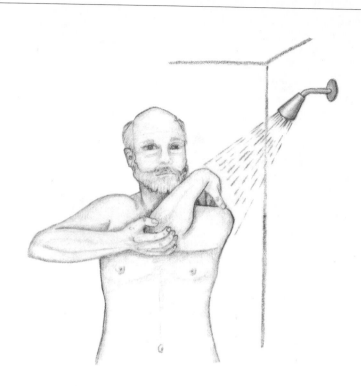

Elbow Across Chest, Left Across

• Grasp the outer side of your left elbow with your right hand, and pull your left arm straight across your chest until you feel tension (but not pain) in the left shoulder blade area. Do not move your hips or back at all. Hold the tense position for about four to six seconds.

• Let go of your left elbow and return to neutral, with your elbow straight out in front. Pull across your chest again, holding for four to six seconds, and then returning to neutral. Repeat four more times for a total of six repetitions.

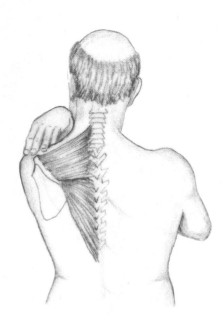

**Left Elbow Across
with Trapezius Muscle**

• Now do the same on the other side. Lift your right hand so that its fingers touch your right shoulder with your right elbow pointing straight out. Grab the right elbow with your left hand and pull your right arm straight across your chest. Hold for four to six seconds.

• Release your arm until your right elbow points straight out again. Pull across your chest and then release five more times, for a total of six repetitions.

- Are you tighter on one side than the other? What do you think causes this? Leaning on a desk while you read? Tight muscles on one side? Think about it! (And look at the posture suggestions in Chapter 10.)

- You can vary the part of the rhomboid muscle exercised by doing this exercise while the elbow is pointed at a 45 degree angle up or down. Experiment — which feels best to you? Or do them all!

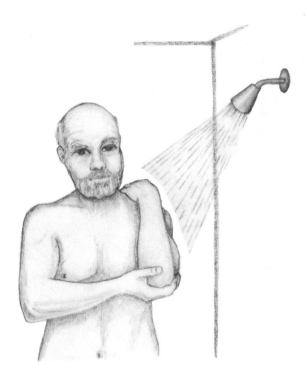

Elbow Down Variation

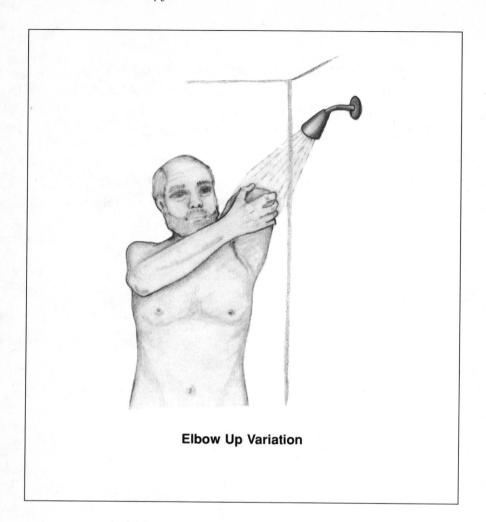

Elbow Up Variation

Exercise 5: Seal to Swan

shower   *middle back*

• Begin in the usual comfortable, erect position.

• Without raising your shoulders or turtling your neck, bring your shoulders straight forward, as though you were trying to touch them in front of you.

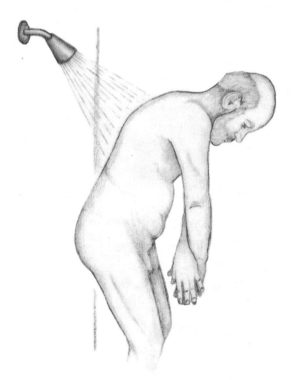

The Seal

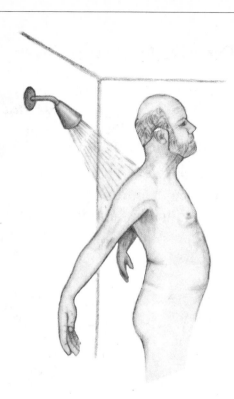

The Swan

• With your arms straight down, cross your wrists in front of you and rotate so you can clap your hands. Bend slightly forward to increase the stretch, and you will look a bit like a trained seal at the circus, clapping its flippers. This will "fan out" your shoulder blades in back, and you will feel tension in the middle back. Try to aim the flow of water right where it's tightest.

• Keep your leg and buttocks muscles as relaxed as possible — they may tend to tighten.

•   Hold the seal position for approximately six seconds.

•   Now, uncross your wrists, letting your shoulders relax. Without raising your hands (or turtling your neck), bring your shoulders straight back and let your hands move gracefully out to the sides and back. This is the serene and dignified posture of the swan. Allow your arms to hang loosely behind you. Don't raise your shoulders to get them further back.

•   Hold this position for about six seconds. You can raise your chin slightly, if that feels more natural.

•   Repeat five times, for a total of six repetitions. It is the movement from seal to swan and back that works both chest and back muscles, but hold each position to feel the stretch. Don't forget to breathe!

Exercise 6: Scared Cat to Swaybacked Horse

*bath or hot tub**   *middle and lower back*

•   Place a towel or special cushion beneath yourself to soften the hard tub bottom.

•   Get down on all fours, with your weight well balanced. The *tops* of your toes should be touching the tub floor. The depth of the water doesn't really matter, as long as you've been soaking before the exercise (and your face is above the surface!).

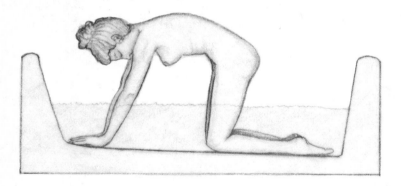

The Scared Cat

* See shower variation, page 74.

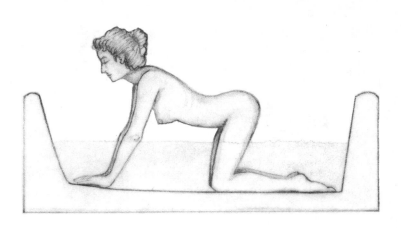

The Swaybacked Horse

• Gently arch your back upwards, like a frightened cat. Let your head drop down, and hold the position for six seconds. Try not to tighten any muscles other than those directly needed to arch the back.

• Slowly and carefully begin to flatten your back, and relax your stomach and back muscles so that the small of your back drops down. At the same time, raise your head as though you were looking at a spot on the wall. This is the swaybacked horse part of the exercise. Hold it for six seconds, and then return to neutral.

• Repeat both positions five times, for a total of six repetitions. If you like, coordinate your breathing with your counting of seconds.

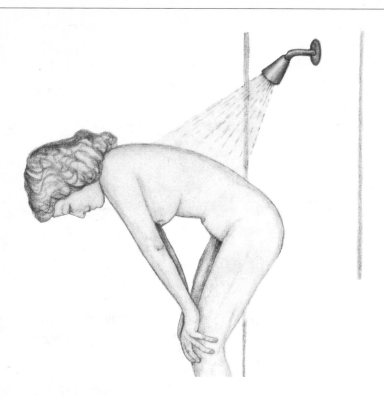

Shower Variation Cat

shower variation:

•   Bend your legs slightly, resting your hands and your weight on your knees. Arch the small of your back upwards, squeezing your stomach in towards your spine, and forming a curve with your head hanging down. Hold for six seconds. This is the scared cat position. Now drop your lower back by relaxing your stomach muscles and letting the curve reverse. With your hands still on your knees, raise your head to form the horse. Hold again for six seconds, directing the spray of water to your middle back.

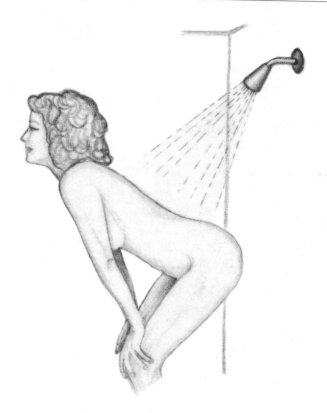

Shower Variation Horse

- Repeat five times, for a total of six repetitions.

Exercise 7: Knee Walk

bath, hot tub   *lower back*

• Position your towel or cushion on the tub floor beneath you. You may want a cushion behind your head and shoulders as well.

• Recline against the back of the tub, or the edge of the hot tub.

• Settle down until you are nearly lying on your back, but don't drown. Your knees should be up, and your feet suspended, loose, and just comfortably dangling.

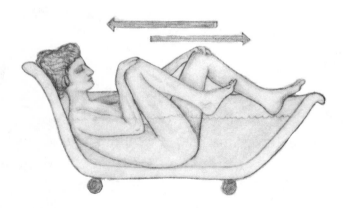

Knee Walk

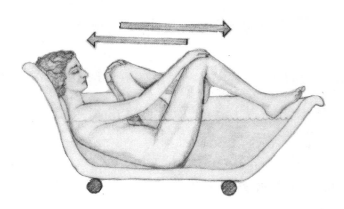

Knee Walk

• Gently place your left palm on your left kneecap, and your right palm on your right kneecap. "Walk" your knees back and forth as illustrated, at whatever speed seems most comfortable to you.

You don't need to move each knee very far — a total of three to five inches back and forth is plenty.

• Do this for 30 to 60 seconds, or for as long as you like. Pay attention to your breathing: keep it calm and regular.

• Once you are comfortable with this exercise, you can walk your knees without using your hands. The knee walk is good for your abdominal muscles, and doing it "no hands" will increase the workout for your stomach. Just let your hands brace your body behind you, or rest on your stomach. But don't overdo it at first, with or without hands, or you'll be sore.

Exercise 8: Knee Circles

bath, hot tub   *lower back*

- Position your towel or cushion beneath you.

- This exercise begins from the same position as Exercise 7, the Knee Walk, lying on your back, with knees up, and your feet comfortably dangling.

- Gently place your left palm on your left kneecap, and your right palm on your right kneecap. Keep your knees tightly together, and your palms on your knees, as you go through this exercise.

- Move your knees in a circular motion, as if you were drawing a plate in the air with them. Move at whatever speed seems most comfortable to you. You can roll a *little bit* from side to side, but try to keep your entire lower back on the tub bottom at all times.

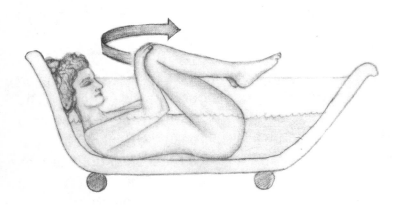

Knee Circles

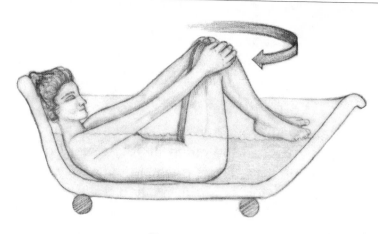

Knee Circles

• You don't need to make big circles at first, or move the knees very far — begin by making a circle about the size of a small plate. Do this for a few seconds at first, and work up to 30 to 60 seconds.

• As with Exercise 7, once you've learned to do the knee circles, you can do them without using your hands. This also is an excellent abdominal exercise. Just be careful not to overdo it, until you've gradually built up some strength in the region.

• Making larger circles will require more muscular strength. Once making small plate circles for 60 seconds is no longer a challenge, start making dinner plates, or even pizza plate motions!

Exercise 9: Pelvic Tilt

shower*   *lower back*

• Stand with your knees bent slightly, hands at your sides. Flatten the curve of your lower back by sucking your stomach in, pressing your belly button back toward your spine, and lifting your pubis up. This is the backward tilt. (Think of the direction your stomach goes in.) Hold for six seconds.

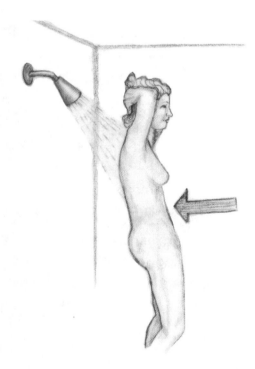

Pelvic Tilt, Backward

* See bath or hot tub variation, page 82.

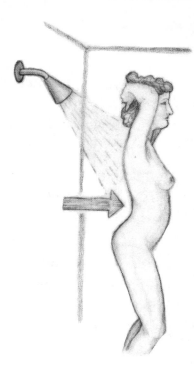

Pelvic Tilt, Forward

• Now relax your stomach and move your buttocks back, curving the small of your back. Your knees are still bent. This is the forward tilt. Hold for six seconds, letting the water spray on your lower back.

• Repeat five more times, for a total of six repetitions.

bath or hot tub variation:

• Begin by lying on your back (using a towel for padding, if necessary), with your knees up and your feet flat on the tub floor. Rest your head against the back of the tub.

• Suck your stomach in so that the curve of your lower back flattens out against the bottom of the tub. Let your pelvis move you as you do this. Hold for six seconds.

• Now let your stomach out and arch your back so that your buttocks push against the floor. Your lower back is slightly curved. Hold this position for six seconds. Don't forget to breathe.

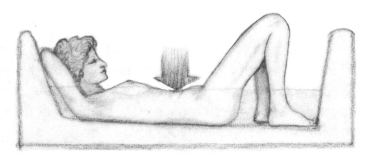

Backward Tilt, Tub Variation

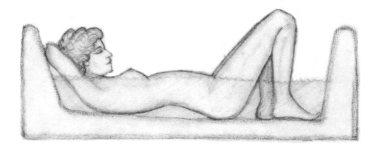

Forward Tilt, Tub Variation

•   Repeat five more times, for a total of six repetitions.

seated variation

•   Yes, do it in a chair. Sit straight up, with your head erect, and tuck your behind under for six seconds. Don't turtle your neck. Then arch your back so that your behind pushes into the back of the chair for six seconds.

7

Stretching Techniques

Why Stretching Works

After an exercise session loosens and flushes out a tight muscle, stretching acts like the final hearty squeeze that you give a sponge after you've wet it and wrung it out repeatedly. This final stretch helps increase the range of motion of a muscle by lengthening muscle fibers and stimulating joints.

The difference, by the way, between the exercises and the stretches of this program can be quite subtle. In an exercise, the motion is repeated, and not held for longer than about six seconds. A stretch might consist of the exact same motion, but done only once, and with the position held motionless for 30 to 60 seconds.

A stretch involves extending the muscle and joint to the extreme position that can be comfortably reached. Although many people think it's healthy to "warm up" by stretching *before* engaging in exercise, in reality, a stretch is best done *after* the body has been warmed up by exercise. That's why the following stretches are always meant to be done last when used in the Hot Water Therapy routines, after relaxation, deep massage, and exercise.

About the Stretches

The stretches are grouped by trouble spot, indicated on the right side of the page. On the left side, you'll see whether a particular stretch is suited to the bath, hot tub, or shower. As with the exercises, Chapter 8 will tell you how to integrate the stretches into the routines. As you test them out, remember that stretches are best done at the end of any routine, when your muscles are warm and loose.

The stretches should *never* hurt. When you approach your final stretch position, you may expect to feel some tightness or tension. As you continue to hold the stretch, the tightness will probably diminish. This is a sign that the muscle fiber is relaxing and stretching. It is *not* an invitation to stretch further — or to bounce. Don't. Next time you do the stretch, you can try a slightly more extreme position. The idea is to find a "just-shy-of-pain" position when beginning the stretch, and to stay with that position — no more — during the rest of that stretch.

Breathing deeply and regularly during a stretch will help to relax you and increase the effectiveness of the stretch. With each breath, feel the healing steam and oxygen rush in, and all stress and tension fly out.

Stretch 1: Head to the Side

shower   *neck, trapezius,*
                                              upper back

• Begin by standing in a relaxed but upright posture. Your head is "hanging from a string," and your
shoulders are like a heavy coat hanging loosely from
a coat hanger.

• Reach over your head with your right hand and
place your right fingers on, under, or just above your
left ear (depending on how far you can comfortably
reach). Your right elbow should be pointing directly
to your right. Don't rest the right arm's weight on the
head. Keep your right arm light as a feather.

• Let the hanging fingers of your left hand "walk"
down the side of your left leg for an inch or so, while
you gently pull your head to the right with your right
fingers.

• Don't overdo this stretch. As soon as you begin
to feel tightness in the left side of your neck, hold the
position for 30 seconds. Don't forget to breathe deeply, and relax into the stretch.

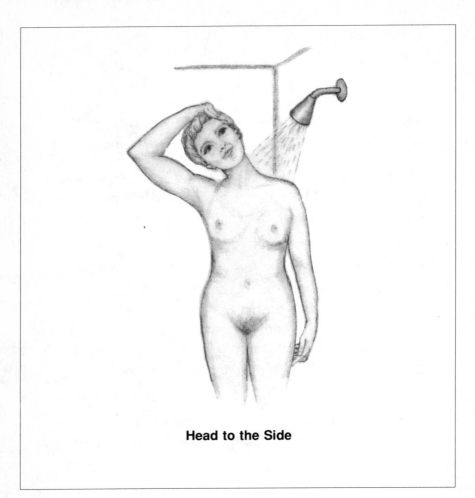

Head to the Side

• Return your head slowly to an upright position, and relax for a moment with your arms at your sides. Now reach over your head with your left hand to your right ear, and inch your right hand down your right leg as you gently pull your head to the left with your left hand. Remember to keep your left arm light as a feather. Stop when you feel tension in the right side of your neck, and hold that position for 30 seconds.

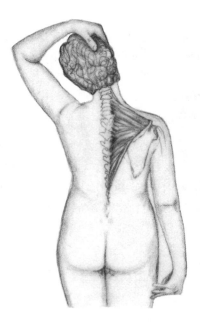

Head to the Side, with Trapezius Muscle

Stretch 2: Head Down

shower   *neck, trapezius,*
                                     upper back,
                                     middle back

•   Stand comfortably, in the "hanging from a string" posture. Keep your shoulders relaxed, and as low as possible.

•   Place the fingertips of both hands at the back part of the top of the head, as though you were peeling off a toupée from the rear forwards. Keep your elbows pointing forward, and don't rest the weight of your arms on your head.

•   Gently begin to press forward with your fingertips, as you drop your chin towards your chest. Continue to press until you feel some tightness, but *not pain*, on both sides of your neck, and perhaps in your upper back.

- Relax into the tightness, and hold the stretch for about 30 seconds. If it should begin to hurt more instead of diminishing, reduce the pressure on your head.

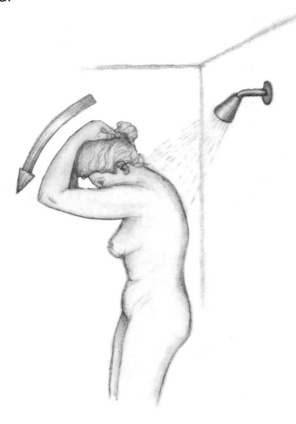

Head Down

Stretch 3: Elbow Across Chest

shower   *middle back*

•   The positions used in this stretch are exactly the same as those used in Exercise 4. The only difference is that you will hold the stretches, both left and right, for 30 seconds each, instead of doing repetitions of six seconds each.

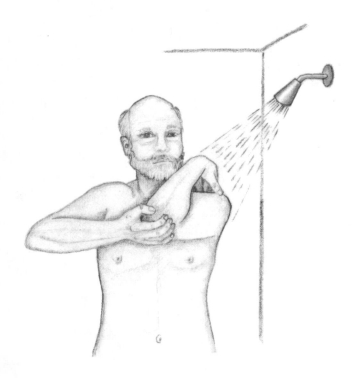

Elbow Across Chest, Left Across

- Begin by standing comfortably, in the erect "hanging from a string" position. Keep your shoulders relaxed and low.

- Touch the fingers of your left hand to your left shoulder, pointing your left elbow straight out from your body at shoulder level.

- Grasp the outer side of your left elbow with your right hand, and pull your left arm straight across your chest until you feel tension (but not pain) in the left shoulder blade area. Do not move your hips or back at all. Hold the tension position for about 30 seconds.

- Return to neutral, letting your arms come to rest at your sides.

- Do the same thing on the other side: right fingers touching right shoulder, right elbow pointing straight out, grab right elbow with left hand and pull right arm straight across chest. Once again, hold for about 30 seconds.

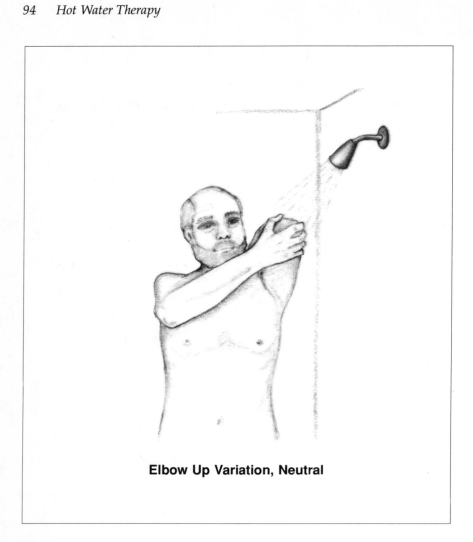

Elbow Up Variation, Neutral

• You can vary the part of the rhomboid muscle exercised by doing this stretch while the elbow is pointed at a 45 degree angle up, or down. Experiment — which stretch feels best to you? Or do them all!

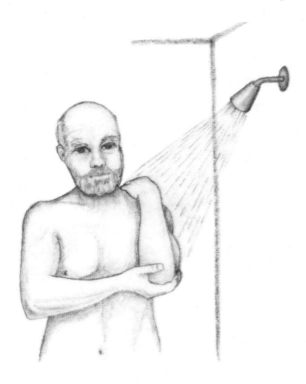

Elbow Down Variation

Stretch 4: Arm Over Head

shower   *middle back*

- Begin by standing up straight, in the "hanging from a string" posture, with your feet approximately shoulder width apart. Your arms and shoulders are loose and low, and your breathing is regular.

- Put your left arm straight above your head, with the elbow nearly but not quite locked, palm forward.

- Grab your left wrist with your right hand, with your right thumb to the front.

- Keeping your left arm straight, and without leaning forward at all, or moving your hips from side to side, pull your left hand across to the right. Don't let your arms move forward — keep them directly overhead as they begin to move to the right. Let yourself begin to bend slightly at the waist.

- In a slow, smooth motion, continue to move your arms, head, and upper back to the right, until you feel tightness in the area under your left arm. Hold this position for 30 seconds.

• Make sure you don't crunch your head down, or turtle your neck. Your neck and head should remain as relaxed as possible, hanging loosely to the right.

• Return gently to neutral, in the standing upright posture. Let your arms hang loose at your sides.

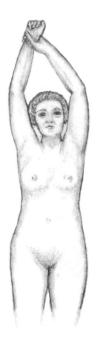

Arm Over Head, Beginning Left Neutral

• Now put your right hand overhead, grasp your wrist with your left hand, and pull across to the left side. Hold this position for 30 seconds.

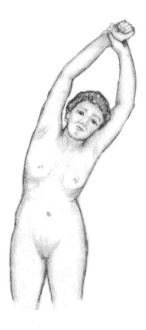

Arm Over Head, Left Stretch

Stretch 5: Seal to Swan

shower   *middle back*

•   The positions used in this stretch are exactly the same as those used in Exercise 5. The only difference is that you will hold the stretch in each position for 30 seconds, instead of doing repetitions of six seconds each.

•   Begin in the usual comfortable, erect position.

•   Without raising your shoulders or turtling your neck, bring your shoulders straight forward, as though you were trying to touch them in front of you.

•   With your arms straight down, cross your wrists in front of you and rotate so you can clap your hands. This is the seal position, as you bend slightly forward and "clap your flippers." Feel your shoulder blades fan out in back, and tension tighten momentarily in the middle back.

•   Keep your leg and buttocks muscles as relaxed as possible — they may tend to tighten.

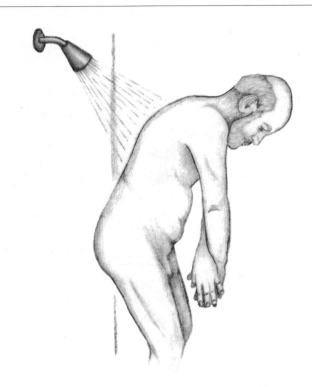

The Seal

• Hold this position for approximately 30 seconds.

• Now, uncross your wrists, and without raising your hands (or turtling your neck), bring your shoulders straight back and let your hands move gracefully out to the sides and back. This is the serene and dignified posture of the swan. Allow your arms to hang loosely behind you. Keep your shoulders low and relaxed.

• Hold this position for about 30 seconds. You can raise your chin slightly, if that feels more natural. Throughout this stretch, direct the water to your upper or middle back; wherever it's needed most. Breathe deeply, and relax.

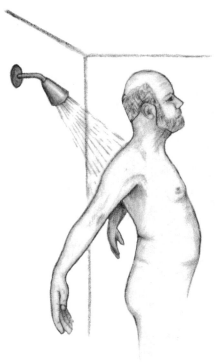

The Swan

Stretch 6: Knee to Chest

bath or hot tub   *middle and lower back*

• You can do this stretch lying down on a towel or cushion in the tub. Begin by setting down in the tub, and making your back as flat as possible against the bottom.

• Bring your left knee up, so that your foot is suspended comfortably, keep your right foot flat on the tub bottom. Raise your left knee high enough to grasp *behind* that knee with either hand, or both. Do *not* grasp the kneecap itself — doing so isn't good for the knee.

• Pull the left knee up as close to the chest as possible. Hold this position for 30 seconds.

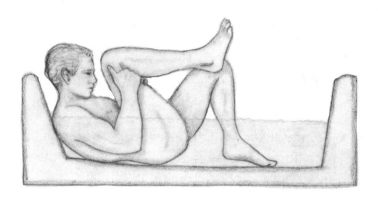

Knee to Chest

• Now lower the left knee slowly, grasp behind the right knee, and raise it to your chest. Try not to move your head or strain your neck while you change sides. Keep your head relaxed and comfortable as you hold for 30 seconds.

• As an advanced stretch, you can begin with both legs stretched out as straight as possible. (Let your feet rest on the tub rim if you run out of room.) Raise one knee to your chest as before, but keep the other leg straight instead of bent. Repeat to the other side after 30 seconds.

Stretch 7: Knee Across

bath or hot tub   *middle and
                                      lower back*

• Begin by lying as flat on your back as possible, with both knees up and both feet flat on the tub bottom. Use a towel or cushion if you like.

• Lift your right leg, and cross it over your left knee, sliding the right knee down as close to the left knee as possible.

• Using the left hand, begin to pull your right knee to the left and slightly down. Keep your pelvis flat on the floor.

• As your knees move to the left and down, feel the stretch on your right side and into the right buttocks. Try to keep your upper back and shoulders flat on the floor of the tub.

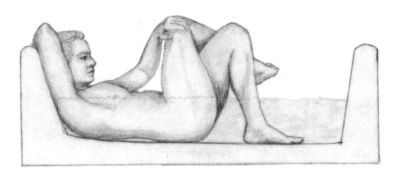

Knee Across, Beginning Stretch to Left

• You will begin to feel this stretch in your lower back. Stop, and hold for 30 seconds, or before it starts to hurt. Remember to breathe as you stretch.

• Now cross your left leg over your right, and use your right hand to pull both legs to the right. Feel the stretch on your left side and buttocks, and hold for 30 seconds.

Stretch 8: Walk to Toes

bath or hot tub   *middle and
                                      lower back*

• Begin in a seated position, with your legs out in front of you. Your knees may be slightly bent, but there should be no more than three or four inches between the bottom of your knees and the tub bottom. You may find it helpful to wet a towel and drape it over your shoulders and back to keep this area under wet heat.

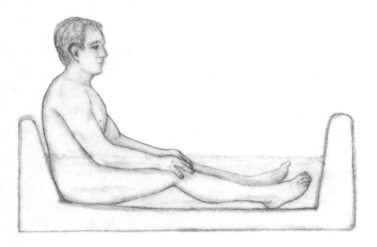

Walk to Toes, Neutral

•   Sit with your back straight, head erect, and your fingertips on your knees. Slowly begin to walk your fingers down your legs towards your ankles. As you lean forward as much as you can from the waist, you may bend your head down if that seems more comfortable. This is a tricky stretch: don't cross that line into pain.

•   Everybody feels this stretch in a different place — some in the neck, some in the upper back, some in the middle back, some in the lower back, some in the legs. Be gentle with yourself.

•   You may not be able to get very close to your toes if your back is tight, as illustrated. That's fine — even a minimal bend will help loosen you up. Just bend until you feel tightness but not pain, and hold the position for at least 30 seconds. With practice, you will be able to hold it for 60 seconds, and move closer to your toes. Try to relax, and breathe deeply.

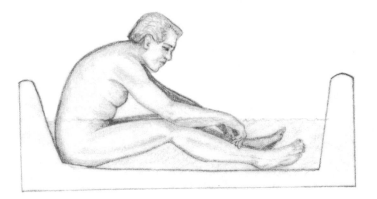

Walk to Toes

towel stretch variation

•   In the unlikely event that you can grab your toes without straining, do so, and then straighten your knees until they lock.

•   If you are among the other 99 percent of people, hold the end of a towel in each hand, and loop the middle of the towel over your toes.

•   This allows you to approximate the toe grab, and to flatten the knees while pulling on the towel. Bend over to whatever extent feels comfortable. Hold for 30 to 60 seconds.

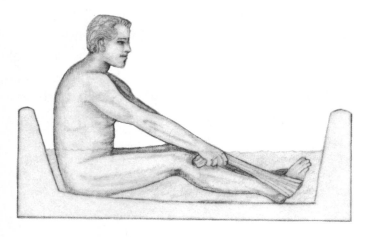

Hamstring Stretch with Towel, Neutral

8

Designing Your Own Routines

About the Routines

Once you have considered all of the massage, exercise, and stretching techniques, the challenge lies in putting them together in ways that will encourage you to use them on a daily basis. To help you do this, this chapter offers suggested full routines, mini-routines, and micro-routines of different types. The suggestions leave room for you to experiment, incorporating the elements that work best for you. Just remember the general guidelines of beginning with relaxation and massage, moving into exercise, and concluding with gentle stretching.

It's best to read through an entire routine and go over it in your head before you begin. Keep the book near your bath...but don't take it into the shower! (One idea is to xerox some pages and put them in a plastic bag or page protector.) As you scan the pictures next to the exercise and stretch descriptions, keep in mind that they do not always demonstrate the entire movement, as they did in the original descriptions. These pictures serve to jog your memory; turn back to the full descriptions for more detail.

The Full Routines

In general, the shower is a better place to do hot water exercises for the upper back and neck areas, and the bath tub a better place to do lower back exercises. Of course, a hot tub is even better than a bath tub, if you're lucky enough to have access to one.

Following are full routines for upper back/neck, middle back, and lower back. Each might take around 10 minutes to complete, or more if you have the extra time to spend on the relaxation and massage parts.

The Full Shower Routine for Headache, Stiff Neck, or Upper Back Pain

• Get in the shower and adjust the water temperature. Concentrate on relaxing and breathing deeply and evenly while the water gently showers onto the back of your neck and upper back. If you need to conserve water, wet a towel thoroughly with warm water and drape it over your back and shoulders. Or you can simply adjust your flow valve. Allow one to three minutes for the soothing benefits of hot water to begin their magic.

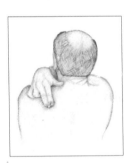

• Staying in the same position, begin to apply deep pressure according to Massage 1, the Trapezius Walk. Make sure to apply gentle pressure to any knotty, tender spots you locate. Continue for one to two minutes.

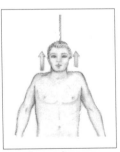

• Begin Exercise 1, Shoulder Lifts, allowing six seconds for each hold. Release the hold slowly, letting your shoulders ease back down into the loose, low neutral position. Rest for a moment, and bring them back up for six seconds. Remember to keep your head high, and "hang from the string!"

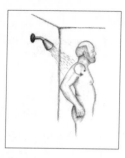

• Do six repetitions of Exercise 2, the Shoulder Circles (three forward and three backward). Take at least 12 seconds to complete each circle.

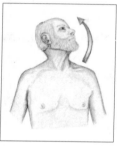

• Do six repetitions of Exercise 3, the Head Rock. Take 12 seconds for each repetition, counting three up, three to neutral, three down, and three back to neutral for each side.

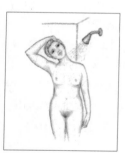

• Finish up with two 30-second repetitions (one to the left, and one to the right) of Stretch 1, the Head to the Side. Visualize yourself relaxing and flushing the muscles of your neck. If you like, incorporate Relaxation 3, Visualization, as an advanced step (described in the next chapter). Remember to breathe!

The Full Shower Routine for the Middle Back

• Get in the shower, adjust the temperature, and spend a few minutes relaxing and breathing deeply.

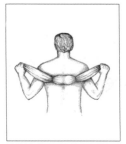

• If you have made the Back-uPressure device, place the balls between the inner edge of your shoulder blade and your spine, and work any tender spots you find by leaning *gently* into the shower wall. Do both sides until any tenderness fades. Allow 15 to 60 seconds per side.

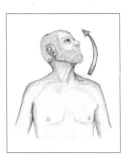

• Turn so that the water is pouring onto your upper back. Do six repetitions of Exercise 3, the Head Rock (three to the left and three to the right). Count six seconds for each up rock and for each down rock.

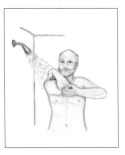

• Do six repetitions of Exercise 4, Elbow Across Chest (three to the left and three to the right). Allow six seconds for each hold, moving gently and rhythmically to and from neutral for another six-count.

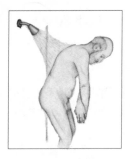

• Do six repetitions of Exercise 5, the Seal to Swan. Do six seconds of seal, followed by six seconds of swan, for each repetition.

• Do Elbow Across the Chest again, but this time as in Stretch 3. Hold the elbow across for 30 seconds, then switch sides and hold for another 30 seconds.

• Finish up with one minute of Stretch 5, the Seal to Swan. After 30 seconds of seal, move gracefully into the swan position and hold for 30 seconds. If you like, use Relaxation 3, Visualization, to visualize yourself relaxing and flushing the muscles of your middle back. Keep your breathing deep and regular.

The Full Bathtub Routine for the Lower Back

• Once the tub is filled with water of the right temperature, climb in and lie down. Breathe deeply in and out in a slow, regular rhythm, letting your body respond to the soothing heat and comfort. As you breathe, picture healing steam and oxygen flowing in, and troubles and toxins washing out. Allow two to four minutes of relaxation time, or more if you like.

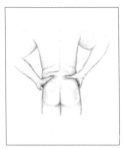

• Sitting upright, do two minutes of Massage 2, the Sacrum Stroke. If you locate any tender points, give them direct pressure treatment until the pain diminishes. If you've made a BackuPressure device, work your lower back with it by leaning against the tub.

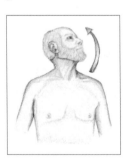

• Sitting upright, do six repetitions of Exercise 3, the Head Rock. Take six seconds for each up rock, and six for each down rock. You may wish to dunk a small towel, and drape it over your neck and shoulders.

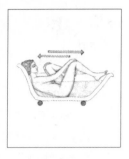

• Settle in the tub, placing a small towel under you if you lack natural padding. Bring your knees up, gently place your palms on your kneecaps and do approximately 30 to 60 seconds of Exercise 7, the Knee Walk.

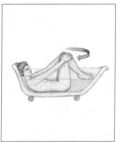

• Put your knees down, feet flat on the floor, and relax for a moment. In fact, you might try a minute of one of the Relaxation Exercises in Chapter 9, if you like. Then settle back down so your entire lower back is flat on the tub bottom. Do 30 to 60 seconds of Exercise 8, the Knee Circles.

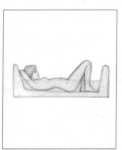

• Now, with your knees still bent, gently lower your feet to the tub bottom. Do six repetitions of Exercise 9, the Pelvic Tilt. Suck your stomach in and press your lower back against the bottom of the tub for six seconds, and then release and arch up for six seconds.

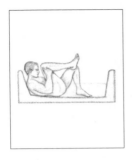

• Go on to the stretches with one minute of Stretch 6, the Knee to Chest, doing 30 seconds for each leg. Remember to grasp behind your knee as you pull your leg to your chest and hold for the stretch.

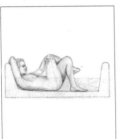

for 30 seconds.

• Do one minute of Stretch 7, Knee Across. With your back straight and low, and your knees bent, cross your right leg over your left knee and pull to the left for 30 seconds. Your pelvis stays flat and centered. Repeat right,

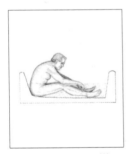

long as you like.

• Sit up higher, and finish off with 30 seconds of Stretch 8, the Walk to Toes. Take as long as you need to walk your fingers down toward your toes, and then count for the hold. When you're done, relax in your bath for as

The Full Hot Tub Routine for the Whole Back

This full routine is a little longer than the others, since anyone with access to a hot tub will probably want to soak in it for as long as possible. Bring a pitcher of cool water with you when you do this one — you can bet you'll sweat.

• Climb in, sit or lie down, and concentrate on relaxing. (If you like, try some of the relaxation techniques from Chapter 9 at this point.) Allow yourself two to four minutes to become completely relaxed.

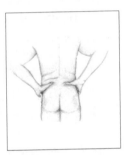

• Do two minutes of Massage 2, the Sacrum Stroke. If you locate any tender points, give them the direct pressure treatment until the pain diminishes. If you've made a BackuPressure device, work your middle back.

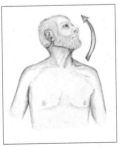

• Sitting upright, do six repetitions of Exercise 3, the Head Rock (three to the left, and three to the right). Allow six seconds for each up rock, and six for each down rock. You may wish to dunk a small towel, and drape it over your neck and shoulders.

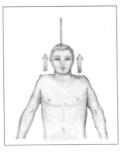

• Still sitting upright, do six repetitions of Exercise 1, Shoulder Lifts. Allow six seconds for each hold, and relax for six seconds in neutral between lifts. (If you prefer, substitute Exercise 2, Shoulder Circles. Or — do both!)

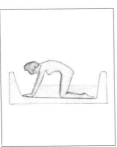

• Get down on all fours, and do six repetitions of Exercise 6, the Scared Cat to Swaybacked Horse. Spend six seconds in the cat position, back arched, and head down, and six seconds in the horse position, back bowed, head up, for each repetition.

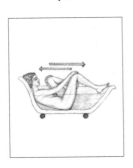

• Lie on your back, bring your knees up, and do 30 to 60 seconds of Exercise 7, the Knee Walk. This exercise works well on the hot tub bench, as does the one above.

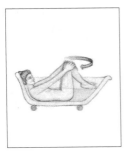

• Let your legs float, and relax for a moment. If you like, do a minute of one of the relaxation exercises from Chapter 9. Then do 30 to 60 seconds of Exercise 8, the Knee Circles, on your back again.

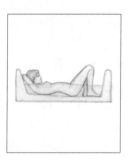

• Now, with your knees still bent, place your feet back on the tub bottom. Do six repetitions of Exercise 9, the pelvic tilt. Allow six seconds for the hold in each position, forward and backward.

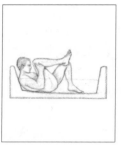

• Go on to the stretches with one minute of Stretch 6, Knee to Chest, doing 30 seconds for each leg. Grasp gently behind your knee as you pull that leg to your chest and hold for the stretch.

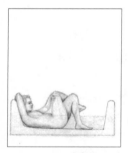

• Do one minute of Stretch 7, Knee Across, spending 30 seconds on each side. Keep your pelvis flat and centered as you cross one leg over the other knee and pull to the side. Stretch, return to neutral, and repeat to the other side.

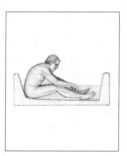

• Sit back up, and finish off with a 30 second hold of Stretch 8, the Walk to Toes. Then relax in the hot tub for as long as you like.

About the Mini-Routines

The mini-routines are short preventative sessions that you can do during a quick shower for your neck, upper, middle, and lower back. It's a great way to start a day, and an efficient use of your time. After all, a few minutes a day in the shower can help you avoid a week-long episode of back pain.

Although having the water cascade soothingly onto your back as you do these mini-routines is very helpful, you can do them dry, as well. Since it's best to integrate the benefits of warm water into all routines, you'll want to read about hot packs at the end of this chapter. They allow you to benefit from Hot Water Therapy even when you're far from a shower or tub.

You won't find mini-routines for the bath tub or hot tub, since anyone with time enough to take a bath or hot tub shouldn't be in too much of a hurry to do a ten-minute full routine!

The following are some suggested mini-routines. If you like, study the relaxations, massage techniques, exercises, and stretches — and make up some mini-routine variations of your own.

A Mini-Routine for the Neck and Upper Back

• Allow yourself thirty seconds to one minute of pure relaxation. If you like, try Relaxation 1 or 2 from Chapter 9.

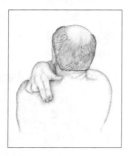

• Now do thirty seconds to one minute of Massage 1, the Trapezius Walk. Work those trigger points! Remember to press gently but firmly into the sore spots until the pain or tension recedes.

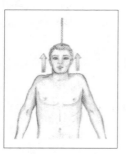

• Do three repetitions of Exercise 1, Shoulder Lifts, allowing six seconds for each hold, and six seconds for rest in neutral for each repetition. Keep that head high (remember to "hang from the string")!

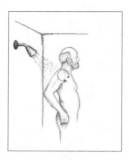

• Do six repetitions of Exercise 2, Shoulder Circles, (three forward, then three back). Allow six seconds for each circle.

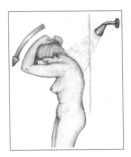

• Finish with 30 seconds of Stretch 2, the Head Down.

Total time: About three minutes!

A Mini-Routine for the Middle Back

• Begin with just a few seconds of relaxation. You might like to try Relaxation 2 from Chapter 9, the breath-counting meditation, for one or two sets of four breaths each.

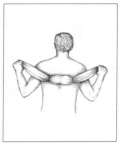

• Do 30 seconds of Massage 1, the Trapezius Walk. Or if you have made a BackuPressure, use the device on your middle back between the spine and the shoulder blades for 30 seconds.

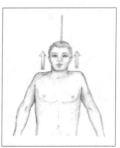

• Do three repetitions of Exercise 1, Shoulder Lifts, holding for six seconds and relaxing between. Keep that head high, and remember to "hang from the string"!

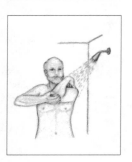

• Do six repetitions of Exercise 4, Elbow Across Chest, three to the left, and three to the right. Allow six seconds for each hold, relaxing and returning to neutral between.

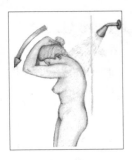

• Do 30 seconds of Stretch 2, the Head Down.

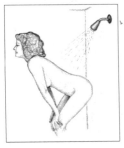

• Finish with one minute of Exercise 6, Cat to Horse, but do it as a stretch. Spend 30 seconds in the cat position, then 30 seconds in the horse position. Remember to breathe.

Total time: Between two and three minutes!

A Mini-Routine for the Lower Back

• Begin with just a few seconds of relaxation. If you like, try Relaxation 1 or 2 from Chapter 9.

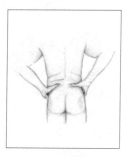

• Now do Massage 2, the Sacrum Stroke, for 30 seconds.

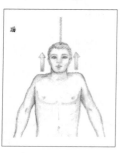

• Do six repetitions of Exercise 1, Shoulder Lifts, holding each lift for six seconds and relaxing and loosening your shoulders between. Keep that head high (remember to "hang from the string")!

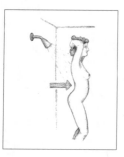

• Do six repetitions of Exercise 9, the Pelvic Tilt (shower variation), three forward and three back. Hold each position for six seconds before changing.

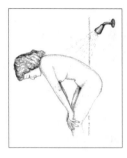

• Now move to Exercise 6, Scared Cat to Swaybacked Horse (shower variation). Do this as a *stretch,* however, holding each position for 30 seconds.

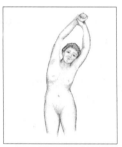

• Finish with one minute of Stretch 4, Arm Over Head, 30 seconds to each side. Don't put any weight on your head as you reach your arm across!

Total time: About four to five minutes!

About the Hot Pack

Wish you had access to a shower, bathtub, or hot tub at the office? Try a homemade hot pack!

A hot pack is a simple device that delivers wet heat to your body. The term usually refers to a waterproof bag filled with wet gel or clay that can be heated and applied to the body. Most pharmacies will have at least a few in stock, of varying sizes.

You can easily make your own hot pack with a kitchen sponge and a hand towel. If you have a microwave, begin by wetting and wringing out the sponge. Fold it inside the hand towel so that the sponge is in the center lengthwise. Now microwave it for 30 seconds. Remove, holding the dry ends of the towel — and be sure to check the heat with your fingertips before applying it to your back.

If you don't have access to a microwave, boil some water in a teapot. Place a sponge on top of a hand towel, and carefully pour a small amount of the boiling water onto the sponge. Now wrap the sponge in the towel securely, so that no part of it is exposed and no boiling water can drip directly out. If the towel itself got very wet, you may want to replace it with a new one. For safety, place a dry towel across your neck or shoulders before applying the hot pack. As the water cools a bit, you may choose to remove the dry towel.

Placing the hot pack on your trouble spot while doing a mini-routine gives you some of the benefits of wet heat when a shower or a bath just isn't practical. It can be draped over the back of your neck, or you can keep it between you and the wall or chair as you do standing or seated pelvic tilts (Exercise 9). You can balance it on your lower back as you do Exercise 6, the Cat/Horse, or place it under you as you do Exercises 7 and 8, the Knee Walk and Knee Circles.

So if you miss your "hot water fix" during the day, try incorporating a hot pack into your daily mini-routines, and turn your dry routines into damp ones!

About the Micro-Routines

These are routines that can be done in just a few seconds, or two minutes at most, anywhere, anytime. Although they don't seem like enough to make a difference, they can have a powerful cumulative effect if you take time to do them even half a dozen times a day (for a total time expenditure of a few minutes).

Following are a few suggestions for micro-routines. Once again, feel free to make up some of your own, using any of the material in this book.

A Micro-Routine for the Neck and Upper Back

• Do 30 seconds of Massage 1, the Trapezius Walk. Work those trigger points!

• Do six repetitions of Exercise 2, Shoulder Circles: three forward, and three back. Take about six seconds to complete each one.

• Do two repetitions of Exercise 3, the Head Rock, counting six seconds for each up and for each down.

• Finish with 30 seconds of Stretch 2, Head Down.

A Micro-Routine for the Middle Back

•   Do four repetitions of Exercise 4, Elbow Across Chest, two with the left elbow, and two with the right. Allow six seconds for each repetition.

•   Do two repetitions of Exercise 5, Seal to Swan. Do six seconds of seal, followed by six seconds of swan, for each repetition.

•   Finish with 30 seconds of Stretch 2, Head Down.

A Micro-Routine for the Lower Back

•   Do 15 to 30 seconds of Massage 2, the Sacrum Stroke

•   Do three repetitions of Exercise 9, the Pelvic Tilt, counting three seconds forward and three back. This can even be done while sitting in a chair, and no one need know you're doing it. Great at long meetings!

•   Do two repetitions of Exercise 6, Scared Cat and Swaybacked Horse (shower variation) as a stretch. Spend 30 seconds in the cat position, and 30 seconds in the horse position, and then repeat.

9

Advanced Relaxation Techniques

About the Relaxation Exercises

Hot water will help your body to relax. Your own mind can help, too. The following relaxation exercises have been adapted from *The New Three Minute Meditator*, by David Harp, with Dr. Nina Feldman (New Harbinger, 1990). These exercises may take a few tries to master. But once you've learned them, you'll be able to utilize them rapidly and effectively.

Relaxations 1 and 2 are probably the best ones to use in the beginning of a routine, and Relaxations 2 and 3 the most useful during a routine. They can be applied to any trouble spot, from head to foot, and used for as long or as short a period as you like. You can incorporate them into routines or use them whenever tension strikes. Either way, once you master them both body and mind will benefit.

Relaxation 1: Progressive Relaxation

This exercise will help you relax your entire body, perhaps more completely than you ever have before. The variation following it will help you create a mental image of this relaxed state that you can recreate instantly whenever you need to. If you have any joint or bone problems, please discuss this exercise with your physician or chiropractor before trying it.

You may find it easiest, in the beginning, to practice this exercise while lying in bed, face up and arms at your sides. Take as long as you need the first few times you do it, probably at least ten or fifteen minutes.

• Make fists with both hands. Really clench your fingers into your palms, although not so tightly as to be uncomfortable. Feel the tightness in your wrists, and even up into your forearms. Hold the tension for five or six seconds, then relax it. Let your hands become heavy and limp.

• Tense your fists again, for a similar amount of time, squeezing until the muscles begin to quiver. Relax again. Feel how heavy and warm your hands are now. Feel the warmth and heaviness travel up through your wrists to your lower arms. Your hands seem to drag everything down: as though they're made of molten lead, warm and soft and very heavy.

• Shift your focus to your upper arms. Tense your biceps, making sure that your hands remain relaxed and heavy. Hold the tension for a few seconds until your arms begin to quiver, and then relax. Your entire arms are heavy and limp. Now tense your arms again — hold — and then release. Feel how heavy everything is, from your shoulders to your fingertips. As warm, and heavy, and soft, as molten lead.

• Perform this same process — tensing and relaxing, then tensing and relaxing — for as many muscle groups as time allows. After doing your arms, try doing your feet, calves, thighs, buttocks, stomach, chest, and shoulders. Then concentrate on your neck, jaw, and eyes. Tense and relax, tense and relax. Warm and heavy, warm and heavy. Try to cultivate as relaxed a feeling as you can, throughout your entire body.

After you've done this exercise a few times, you'll find yourself able to feel relaxed without needing to do as much tensing and relaxing. You'll become expert at distinguishing between tense muscles and relaxed muscles, and you'll be able to focus in on areas that most need relaxation help. As you practice this exercise, remember that feeling of tension melting away; it will help you visualize real relaxation any time you're under stress or ready to begin a routine. For more ideas on visualization, see Relaxation 3. You'll also find a visualization variation to use with *this* exercise at the end of the chapter.

Relaxation 2: Breath Counting Meditation

This exercise will help you quiet your mind by stilling the constant mental chatter that flows through it. Doing so will train you to focus your mental attention more skillfully, and enable you to become more aware of physical and mental stress before it reaches an uncontrollable level.

•   Begin by practicing this meditation while sitting comfortably in a quiet place. Then simply *count* the exhale of each breath, mentally: "Inhale...1, Inhale ...2, Inhale...3, Inhale...4." After four complete breaths, begin again with "Inhale...1." Strive not to lose your count, and also not to alter or regularize your breathing in any way. Try to feel the physical sensation of each breath, both inhale and exhale, as it passes through your nose or mouth.

•   If you find yourself thinking about *anything* except the feel of your breath and the number of that breath, return to focus on the sensation of breathing, and on the number of that breath. If you are not absolutely sure what number breath you're on, begin again with "Inhale...1." No judging, no "I blew the count" thoughts, just back to "Inhale...1."

Right now, consider the breath focus and count to be your "preferred" thoughts. Thoughts of lunch, memories, or other intruders will just be gently replaced by "Inhale…1, Inhale…2" and so on, *as soon as you notice them* creeping in. And they will! Of course it's difficult to stay focused, but with practice, it gets easier and easier.

• After you've meditated for a few moments, you may want to direct your attention momentarily away from the breath, and towards any part of your body. Is it tight? Relaxed? In pain? Where exactly is the pain?

Once you feel comfortable doing this meditation for a few minutes at a time, try doing it *while* you do the exercises and stretches of Chapters 7 and 8. If the exercise or stretch seems to bring up tense or somewhat painful sensations, just keep breathing and counting, breathing and counting, as you relax into the sensation. (You'll be counting for most exercises anyway; why not try to coordinate these counts with your breathing? It's okay if your "seconds" become a bit longer as you count!) Keeping your mind relaxed can help your body relax as well.

Relaxation 3: Relaxed Muscle Visualization

A tremendous amount of evidence indicates that after you've spent some time clearly visualizing or imagining yourself performing an activity, it becomes easier for you to do it in real life. This technique works in almost any sphere, from athletics to music to relaxation, and the key element seems to be the degree of "real-ness" of the visualization. So it clearly pays to spend some time practicing and strengthening this most useful skill.

In a way, the term *visual*ization is a bit of a misnomer, since this technique's effectiveness is increased when senses other than the visual can be incorporated into every exercise. In the following exercise, try to re-create in your mind a vivid sense of sight, feel, smell and taste.

Picture a lemon in your mind's eye, as clearly as possible. As yellow as the sun, its thick skin minutely wrinkled, and just a touch oily to the hand. Dig your fingernail into the peel, and see a tiny spray of citric oil arch out into the air. Pull some peel off, to expose the white fibers covering the juicy, wet, pulpy insides.

You smell the tartness as you bite deep into the lemon, and taste the sourness. The saliva leaps into your mouth.

If you were able to visualize the lemon with any clarity, you probably salivated even before you imagined biting into it. And that's the point of this body-mind exercise.

Most people would consider salivation to be a bodily process outside of their conscious control. And yet we salivate when we think of lemons. Just the thought of the taste of citrus somehow stimulates a gland in the mouth to produce a secretion.

Practice your visualization with this lemon exercise. Can you "train" your salivary glands to spring into action at the first thought of a lemon? At the word "lemon"?

Practice visualizing a tight muscle relaxing, its tiny fibers lengthening and becoming less dense. Visualize the blood surging in, bringing life-giving oxygen and washing away wastes. Use this, or a visualization of your own creation, during the exercise and stretching portions of your routines for added effectiveness and enjoyment.

Progressive Relaxation With Visualization: A Combination

After you've practiced Relaxation 1 and Relaxation 3 a few times, try combining the two! Once you feel really relaxed using Progressive Muscle Relaxation, savor the warmth and heaviness for a few minutes. Then imagine yourself in a very peaceful place, a place that you associate with relaxation. Try to develop as clear a mental picture as possible of this place, including the way it feels, sounds, looks, smells, and even tastes. Memorize as many details as you can. Perhaps you'd like to visualize a lovely tropical beach. Feel the warm sun, the cool breeze, and the sand under you as you look up at the waving palm fronds. Hear the waves crash, and smell, almost taste, the salt spray in the air.

If you prefer, you may wish to visualize a delightful warm bath, with the feel of the water, the smell of the soap, the sound of the water gently splashing. Since you will sometimes be doing this relaxation exercise in your bathtub, this should be an easy one to visualize!

Hold onto this idea of a special place, even when you're not in the middle of a routine. Just a few seconds' concentration on sun, trees, or *whatever* can give you an instant vacation when stress takes hold. Feel your muscles relax and your mood become sunny without budging an inch. You'll return to face the demands of the moment relaxed and refreshed.

10

Lasting Relief

Helpful Hints For Avoiding Problems...*Before* They Happen

You already know that an ounce of prevention is worth a pound of cure. But somehow, when your back isn't hurting, it's easy to forget how important it is to keep it that way. So you sit for lengthy periods in uncomfortable chairs, and hold the phone between your shoulder and your ear, no hands. You lift heavy objects without bending your knees, and play touch football on the weekends, without exercising gently and then stretching to warm up.

Then, the day after, as your back and neck and sundry joints ache, you wish that you had observed just a few preventive precautions, like the ones that follow.

Lifting

You've heard it before, but it's true: *always* bend your knees and crouch down to pick up something from floor level. Never lean over from the waist to grab it. That's a sure way of putting tremendous stress on your lower vertebrae. And once you're carrying something heavy, hold it in close to you, at waist level, for minimum back stress.

The Phone

A convenient way to ruin your neck is to hold the phone between your head and shoulders so that you can talk "no hands." If you've got to do that often, invest in a lightweight mouthpiece headset that attaches like a hat, or else get a speakerphone.

Desk Work

If you do much deskwork, make sure to take plenty of breaks to exercise and stretch your neck and upper back. Don't remain in the same position for long and only cross and uncross your legs at the knee. You might try placing a box or small stool under your feet to elevate your knees above your hips. It will also help if you keep the lower part of your buttocks or lower back pushed against the back of your chair by doing periodic seated pelvic tilts. Also helpful are frequent Head to Side, Head Down, and Elbow Across Chest stretches.

Driving Too Much

Take frequent breaks to get out and stretch, and try to work in pelvic tilts while you drive. Keep the seat as far forward as is comfortable, to elevate your knees. Do modified head rock exercises while you drive, and shoulder lifts and circles. Just be sure to keep your eyes on the road!

Getting Out of Bed

Instead of keeping your legs flat on the bed, and straining the muscles of your lower back to bring your torso to an upright position — consider the alternatives. Try turning onto your side, with your knees close to the edge of the bed. Place the palm of your upper hand behind your upper knee, then ease your legs over. The weight of your legs will pull you up. You may want to use your other hand on the bed to help push you up.

Yo! Weekend Warriors!

A word of advice: don't. Don't expect to be able to play active sports during the weekend without preparing for it during the week. The way to prepare for it, of course, is to do the routines! If you know that a touch football game with the old gang is likely to be suggested after the reunion, spend a few extra minutes with the routines for the whole week preceding the get-together. And make sure to do a full routine, or at least a mini-routine, as close to the start of the game as is convenient.

When Will You Feel Better?

Most back problems are the culmination of days, weeks, months, or even years of abuse or neglect. You may not even know that you are hurting yourself by wedging that phone between the neck and shoulder, or by sitting for hours without a break at a computer terminal. When back pain happens it may feel sudden and intense, but it may have been building for quite some time. The hot water routines in this book can effectively intervene with many common back problems. For others, the discomfort will be relieved a little bit at a time, day by day or week by week.

As long as you feel some improvement, persevere with the routines until you are able to "manage" the sore or painful areas. Chances are help will come from *your daily routine*, which will also work to keep the discomfort from returning. For the average tight and tender back problem, relief will come within several days to one week. Persevere!

If Hot Water Therapy does not alleviate your back problem, or seems to make it worse, one of several possibilities may be occurring. You may, for instance, be too aggressive with your stretches or pressure point massages. Remember that you never want to cross the line into pain at any time. Be gentle and listen to your body! The point of the hot water routines is to stimulate circulation, loosen tight tissues, and relax taut muscles. If you overdo it, the result of a routine may be further irritation.

Also, Hot Water Therapy is designed as a soft tissue intervention to break a pain cycle. It is not a substitute for professional care of serious back problems. If your pain is severe, radiates to another area (such as down the leg), and involves muscle weakness, you may have pressure on a nerve requiring professional medical attention. Or if a joint becomes irritated, and cannot be relieved with attention at home, it's time to make an appointment with your chiropractor, physical therapist, osteopath, or medical doctor.

Following car accidents, it is generally a good idea to seek out professional help. You can't always tell at the time of the accident how badly hurt you are. Many times, within a few days, people begin to develop pain. When this type of pain is left untreated, it can lead to chronic problems—problems that can be avoided with proper treatment. Also, if an injury or